Guatemala: A Cry From The Heart sends a message that must be heard in Congress and by the American people. It is impossible not to be moved by the Guatemalans whose voices tell of a long history of repression by the military of that country. Mr. Schwantes has done us a great service by helping us hear those voices.

Senator Tom Harkin
United States Senate

An engrossing story. A well-researched, believable look at life in a very troubled country. Schwantes is a keen observer whose concern for the poor shines through his almost journalistic style of writing. For those who wish to be well-informed about Guatemala, it is required reading.

Miriam Showalter, Professor Emeritus
Roosevelt University, Chicago

David Schwantes helps us understand that there is a connection between "them" and "us,"—a personal, powerful, undeniable connection that is historical, economic, ecological, and moral. Their problems truly are our problems, and tough talk backed by military operations won't solve these problems.

Joel Mugge, Executive Director
Center for Global Education, Minneapolis

Excellent insight and amazing sensitivity to the suffering and feelings of the Guatemalan people. David Schwantes reflects a deep Christian commitment. This book is a real contribution.

Missionary in Guatemala

The author sees how the realities of human rights violations especially affect the poor. His reflections reinforce the imperative to implement the universal declarations of human rights in their totality.

Alice Zachmann, SSND
National Coordinator, Guatemala Human Rights Commision/USA
Washington, D.C.

A thoughtful and thought-provoking personal account of a first encounter with the reality of Guatemala. This very readable book will be especially useful to those who seek an introduction to that country, and want to know why we should care about it.

Susan Wood, Executive Director
North American Congress on Latin America (NACLA)
New York City

Particularly unique and compelling because it is written by a businessman who was deeply touched by his personal experience. Anyone who reads this book can never again pretend not to understand the plight of the campesino.

Joe Wierschem, Deacon
Holy Name Parish, Wayzata, Minnesota

A testimony of personal change—spoken through the voice and experience of the Guatemalan people.

Kay Studer, National Coordinator
Women for Guatemala, Concordia, Kansas

This former senior officer of a multinational corporation confronts Third World realities in Guatemala as he had not been able to with his prior business trips. The experiences shared in this book softened his heart and informed his mind, and will have the same impact on the reader.

Don Irish, Professor Emeritus
Hamline University, St. Paul

David Schwantes's book gives us the opportunity to meet, in a highly personal way, Guatemalans from a wide variety of sectors. He presents the facts of the case simply, powerfully, and most importantly, in the words of the Guatemalan people themselves.

Joe Gorin
National Coordinator, Network In Solidarity With The People Of Guatemala (NISGUA), Washington, D.C.

A powerful learning experience on a critical subject—the realities and struggle of Guatemalan life.

Pam Costain, Executive Director
Central American Resource Center, St. Paul

" 'Tis a gift to be free; 'Tis a gift to come down where you ought to be." [From a Shaker song.] David Schwantes understood himself to be free and in the right place until he visited Guatemala, whose people, history and present reality challenged his idea of freedom and his confidence that he was where he ought to be. To read this book is to share his journey, and to be challenged about our own.

Jan Mathison
Augsburg College, Minneapolis

Guatemala

A CRY FROM THE HEART

V. David Schwantes

Health Initiatives Press / Minneapolis

Published in the United States by:

Health Initiatives Press
POB 335
Minneapolis, MN 55331

Library of Congress Catalog Number: 89–82365

ISBN 0–9625066–3–X

Acknowledgments

A few friends—David Duclos, Ray Kosak, Peggy Robertson, Miriam Showalter, and Ray Stock—suffered through the partially completed first drafts of this book and deserve thanks for their feedback and patience.

C. C. Graham and Charlie Sugnet offered helpful insights that moved the project forward. Father Greg Schaffer, Professor Donald Irish, and Kay Studer helped a great deal in the project's later stages. The staff of the Central American Resource Center in St. Paul, Minnesota, were wonderfully supportive, especially Pam Costain.

Deacon Joe Wierschem and his wife, Louise, were indispensable throughout the effort. We met for breakfast one morning before I went to Guatemala and they told me that the most moving experience they had on one of their own recent trips to Central America was when a priest asked them a simple question—"Who is your God?" I thought a great deal about exodus as I traveled, studied, and wrote—about the need we all have to move from the traps of our lives to the fulfillment of our potential. Those thoughts finally led me back to the First Commandment—"I am the Lord your God, who brought you out of the land of Egypt, out of the house of bondage"—and back to my breakfast with these two beautiful people.

To the Center for Global Education and its marvelous staff, my lifelong gratitude for having provided an experience that helped me rediscover values that I had neglected and a First Commandment that had lost some of its priority.

Our guide from the Center, whose name I've been asked not

5

to mention, and my fellow travelers helped make a difficult journey become a time of growth. A special thank you to Mary, our guide in Guatemala, who demonstrated clearly that strength and compassion are compatible.

Five courageous human beings have dedicated their lives to their Guatemalan neighbors. In many ways, this book is their story. That they took time to visit with us was a privilege. It is indicative of the realities of Guatemala that I cannot reveal the names of two of them. But to them, and to Maria Emilia Garcia, Padre Andres Giron, and Father John Goggin, I extend my wishes for safe passage and God's blessings.

Three other meetings, which are described in the book, provided important insight as well. To the two officials of the U.S. embassy, to Arnoldo Baetz Caal of the office of Guatemalan president Vinicio Cerezo, and to Juan Fernando Bendfelt, a director of the private sector organization FUNDESA and a member of the board of regents of the Marroquin University, my sincere thanks.

My thanks also to Ellen Hawley. Her editing brought life and strength to my text. Her endurance and skill were the key to making a collection of words into a book worth reading.

This book was a difficult project, and as always, my wife and family were there to support me every step of the way. It was probably even more difficult for them. I shall always be indebted to them for their kindness during this effort.

I owe thanks to many other people, new friends and old — people who picked me up when I needed that, and people who urged me on when it seemed no one cared.

In some respects this book fulfills a promise. I talked to a young health promoter in the remote mountains of Guatemala one night, a man who constantly put his life at risk by trying to help his friends and neighbors. He asked, "Whom will you tell?" I promised I would tell as many people as I could. I must acknowledge his extraordinary inspiration, and I pray that I've fulfilled my promise to him and to the people of Guatemala.

V. David Schwantes
January 1990

And they were utterly astounded,
for they did not understand about the loaves,
but their hearts were hardened.

Mark 6:51–52

Contents

Guatemala

A CRY FROM THE HEART

Success is a word for which
there could be a thousand definitions.

A great many people equate success with money.
The fact is that there are
millions of affluent "failures"
and an equal number of "successes"
who have nothing in the bank.

One definition of success is:
to win the respect of intelligent persons
and the affection of children;
to earn the approval of honest critics
and endure the betrayal of false friends.

To appreciate beauty,
to find the best in others
and to have accomplished a rescued soul.

To have played and lived with enthusiasm
and seeing with exultation,
to know that even one life has breathed easier
because you have lived.

This is to have succeeded.

"Sanibel Success Story"
Souvenir, Sanibel Island

Introduction

"What d'ya wanna go there for?" the man in the hardware store asked me when I told him I was going to Guatemala. "We've got enough problems right here." We had been talking about the growing epidemic of drugs and violent crime in Minnesota, and about the homeless. It seemed to offend him when I switched gears and began to talk about Central America. Why did I want to go to Guatemala? I went to Guatemala at least in part for adventure — to do something new and exciting. I found adventure all right, but it wasn't the kind I expected.

I had wanted to go to Central America for a long time, but not just as a tourist. I wanted to get close to the people. I wanted to find out what was really happening, and get beneath the veneer of the business and tourist world. With a small group led by guides from the Center for Global Education, I had the chance.

I had traveled to the Third World before, but always as a businessman, glimpsing reality out of the corner of my eye as I hurried to my next meeting. I didn't think dining with bankers had given me a complete perspective on Third World realities, and I wanted to get a closer look.

What I experienced shook my world. I had served the god of money as faithfully as any other god. In Guatemala, I learned anew that there is a huge difference between money and wealth.

Shortly after I returned from Guatemala, my wife and I were invited to a friend's home for holiday desserts. Several tables were filled from end to end and side to side with sumptuous cakes, pies, and dessert creations. Before each was a card noting the name of that particular delight.

Conversation at the party was about holiday ski trips or vacations to sunshine and beaches, or about the latest corporate takeover, with special attention to the Kolberg, Kravis raid on R.J.R. Nabisco.

What made the evening difficult for me was that three nights earlier I had stayed with a peasant family on a mountainside in remote Guatemala. Our dinner was a few tortillas, some beans, and a cup of weak coffee. We slept on the dirt floor of a hut whose walls were made of cornstalks tied together. Reentering my old life was difficult.

In early 1989—a few months after my return from Guatemala—I turned to the writing of this book. I had been a financial officer of a multinational corporation, and more recently I had managed a manufacturing company. Now I sat with a word processor trying to answer the simple question asked by my friend in the hardware store: What d'ya wanna go there for? It was an answer I felt a strong need to discover, and share, as I felt a need to share many of the things I had learned and experienced in Guatemala.

The real importance of my visit to Guatemala wasn't so much finding out about Guatemala, it was finding out about the United States. And it was finding out about myself. The trip and the year of study, writing, and interviewing people who know about Guatemala was not exactly life-changing. But it was life-clarifying.

In some ways I had been hard-hearted. As is typical of the times, I was always busy. This book isn't a romantic story of a bad person who becomes good. But I did make important discoveries, and I did get back to some basic values and feelings I had neglected. As I traveled through Guatemala, my heart softened minute by minute, experience by experience, lesson by lesson.

I had been conservative, personally and politically. For a time I was the chairman of the Republican party in my state senatorial district. Now I believe politics, defined narrowly, are just part of the answer.

The larger need is for people to find more time for each other.

With softened hearts, people can find that time and can reduce the impact of the deadly *D*'s—distancing and denial. Softened hearts can open the way to prayer, and to the stewardship needed in this world and in our own lives.

Central America is changing, and more change is to come. I learned that we can no longer take that region for granted. We must develop new theories, attempt new initiatives, and begin new relationships. Their problems are *our* problems.

———————

Look at the birds of the air:
they neither sow nor reap nor gather into barns,
and yet your heavenly Father feeds them.
Are you not of more value than they?
And which of you by being anxious
can add one cubit to his span of life?

And why are you anxious about clothing?
Consider the lilies of the field, how they grow;
they neither toil nor spin;
yet I tell you, even Solomon in all his glory
was not arrayed like one of these.

But if God so clothes the grass of the field,
which today is alive and tomorrow is thrown into the oven,
will he not much more clothe you,
O men of little faith?

Matthew 6:24–33

———————

The liberal goal of eradicating the squalor
that breeds revolution is valid enough.

Of course, all the money in the world
would be a poor investment
in corrupt, feudal economies.

But the means that have been applied
to easing poverty so far
have been totally inadequate;
whatever the failings of the U.S.,
it cannot be accused of profligacy
toward Latin America.

Strobe Talbot,
TIME *magazine,*
August 8, 1983

1

Desaparecidos

Military Patrols

We arrived in Guatemala City on Monday night, November 21, 1988. The airport was new, impressive, and well equipped. The taxi ride to Zone One, where we were to stay, took us past modern hotels and office buildings, all well lighted and beautifully landscaped.

As we approached our hotel, The Colonial, a modest, comfortable inn near the National Palace, I was struck by the number of military personnel patrolling the streets. They were everywhere, and all of them were heavily armed.

Each patrol had at least four soldiers, and many had more. They were wearing various uniforms, but all of them seemed to be patterned after uniforms I'd seen in the U.S. military. On each block I saw several foot patrols, and these were supplemented by patrols traveling in jeeps—two or three jeeps to a patrol.

There was nothing relaxed about the conduct of the soldiers. They were alert, and acted as if they wanted to make sure everyone was aware of their presence. I thought they had angry eyes.

That night, in our hotel, our guide spelled out the ground rules of the tour, and what she said added to the discomfort I had already begun to feel when I saw the military patrols. We were to take our exposed film, notes, itineraries, agendas, and tape recordings with us at all times, she said. Our hotel might be searched, and if these items were left behind they might be confiscated.

We were not in danger, she said, but many of the people we

would be meeting with were at risk, and the information we recorded could be dangerous to them. We might be followed, and we should be careful in our conversations. We should not use the word *guerrilla* in our conversations, nor should we use the names of neighboring countries. She suggested that we develop code names, and so Nicaragua became Montana, and so on. But we weren't very good at this kind of thing, and our conversations took on the tone of a bad television spy program, providing us with a few welcome moments of comic relief when the absurdity of the situation struck us. But these comic moments were rare. The situation was new to us, and disturbing.

We were told that our telephone calls would be monitored, and the next day, when my wife called from Minnesota, she and I had the most awkward conversation of our twenty-four-year marriage.

Our guide told us that she would translate in the meetings that were scheduled, but that she did not want her picture taken at any time. She explained that this was for her security as well as for the security of the people we would be meeting. She asked us not to use her name, but to refer to her as "a North American living in Guatemala," which we soon condensed to Mary.

It was an embarrassing but characteristic demonstration of our naivete or our hardheadedness that, a few minutes into our first meeting, group members began taking pictures of her despite her request. Thereafter, the group leaders scrambled to find other translators so that Mary could remain as anonymous as possible.

Within hours of arriving in Guatemala, therefore, my experiences were disquieting. The military patrols were too numerous, too well armed, too crisp and intimidating. And although our guide's warnings seemed like something out of a television fantasy, they still disturbed me.

Grupo de Apoyo Mutuo

I began to understand how realistic our guide's caution was when, the next afternoon, we visited the Mutual Support Group (in Spanish, *Grupo de Apoyo Mutuo*, or GAM). There I learned the meaning of a new word, *desaparecido* —a person who has disappeared.

GAM was organized in 1984 by several women who had suffered the loss of a husband or a son to the country's political violence. The women found each other while searching for their loved ones in city morgues, and in other places of death and detention, and they dedicated the organization to helping other families recover their disappeared, and to preventing further violence and demanding punishment for those responsible. The organization now has some three thousand members and wide support, both within Guatemala and internationally.

For a long time, GAM was the only outspoken advocate for human rights in Guatemala. While other organizations plotted strategy and waited until it was safe to operate openly, GAM marched and protested and denounced.

Most reports estimate that forty thousand Guatemalans have disappeared in the last dozen years. Some people believe the number is much higher. The term *desaparecido* has come to be used as both a noun and a participle in Guatemala. One speaks of "the disappeared" and of people who have "been disappeared."

To join GAM is to place oneself in danger. Many of its leaders have been tortured and killed: Hector Gomez Calito and Rosario Godoy de Cuevas, along with her brother and her two-year-old son, are noteworthy examples. GAM supporters and members of their families are frequently abused, tortured, or killed. Some simply disappear.

Canadian Escorts

GAM's office consisted of a few rooms, furnished like the working area of many small businesses: a few tables, files, some outdated office equipment. The walls needed painting and were decorated with posters, slogans, and a few remembrances of GAM members who had become victims of the violence. From the doorway, we had a full view of Pacaya, a volcano that stands majestically near Guatemala City.

At one point, I wandered upstairs, where I was greeted by three students from Canada. They told me they were there to serve as escorts for the GAM leaders, going wherever the leaders went. They did this in the hope that it would keep the leaders alive. In the worst case, the students could serve as witnesses if more leaders were disappeared. The students did not consider themselves beyond danger.

Our meeting room had no tables or chairs. We sat on the dusty floor or leaned against the walls. The dust was not a matter of housekeeping. Dust is a fact of life in Guatemala City's poor neighborhoods—there is nothing to be done about it. Dust and smog choke the lungs throughout the city.

A director of GAM, Maria Emilia Garcia, led the discussion. A young Guatemalan man joined her, and Mary translated.

Maria Emilia Garcia

Maria is the mother of one of the disappeared, Edgar Fernando Garcia, and a founder of GAM. On February 18, 1984, a car with police license plates intercepted Fernando's car as he was on his way to work. He had told his wife that he would return home for lunch, but he didn't.

That evening when he still hadn't returned, his wife called Maria to come and wait with her. At three A.M., men with weapons came to the Garcia home. They shot open the gate and forced their way inside. They went into the kitchen to make themselves coffee. They told the women they had Fernando, and they had his Marxist-Leninist books. They joked about having shot him in the leg.

For three days Maria and her daughter-in-law waited for further word. Then they realized that what had happened to so many others had happened to them: Fernando had been disappeared.

She told us about looking for Edgar in detention centers and in morgues. She told us about seeing there the many bodies of the disappeared.

"But it was never possible to find out his whereabouts," she said. "We know perfectly well that he was taken by members of the army, because the people who were nearby when it happened said that the men who took him were dressed as military police. They put him in a car and they took him away. And so it's been very difficult, because we've never had any news of him since the time he was disappeared."

The room was stone silent.

"I'll share with you one recent case," she said, her voice steady and soft.

"On the first of November, Eliodoro Ordon Camey—he's from the town of San Martin Jilotepeque, in the department of Chimaltenango—that day he went to visit his town, because here the custom is that on the first of November, you go and leave flowers for the dead. So he went to his town to leave flowers for his dead relatives."

When Ordon Camey got to Jilotepeque, the military asked him for his papers, which showed that he now lived in Guatemala City. He was taken to the military base in Chimaltenango, questioned, and released. He was warned never to return to his home village. From his papers, the military knew where he lived, and where he worked.

"On the sixteenth of this month," Maria said, "he left his house at seven-thirty in the morning for work, and he was captured by men dressed as civilians and heavily armed. They put him in a gray car. The family members know what happened because his thirteen-year-old son was with him."

The son reported his father's kidnapping, and the family came to GAM. Witnesses had the car's license plate number, and knew that the kidnappers were military. GAM immediately sent telegrams to President Cerezo and to government ministers asking that they investigate who had taken him, so that he could be found and freed quickly. They filed a writ of habeas corpus with the supreme court and placed advertisements in the press. International support groups denounced the disappearance.

"But, unfortunately, today his body was found," Maria said. Now I understood why, when we entered the office, we had seen several women crying in another room. "He'd been shot, and his body had been thrown close to where his house is. He leaves six children without a father. The oldest is thirteen. The youngest is eight or nine months old."

She paused, breathing deeply and exhaling slowly. It was a long minute before she could speak again. "So that's why we're very worried about this wave of violence that is affecting Guatemalan families so heavily. These are very humble and poor people. They live in very lamentable conditions, and the only support for the family is the man. This man's wife is very upset because, in addition to having her husband kidnapped and now killed, she doesn't know what she's going to do in order to support her family.

"This is just one of thousands of cases. It's truly sad that the leaders of our country leave and go to other countries and say that human rights are respected here in Guatemala, when we here are living the exact opposite."

Ineligible for Service

There was another long pause. We sat quietly on the dusty floor. Then Maria talked about two young men from El Quiche, who came to the capital to see their congressional representative. They had an appointment, and planned to ask for permission not to serve in the civil defense patrols.

"But in the afternoon, people came to take them out of the little hotel where they were staying," Maria said. "They were also dressed as civilians but heavily armed, and outside they had a car that belonged to the police. They took them out by force and forced them into the car."

Six days later the men's relatives came to the city looking for them. They came to GAM, and GAM went through the same series of actions on their behalf as it had for Ordon Camey.

Maria reached into her pocket and produced a telegram that she had received from the director of information of the Defense Department. It said, "Informing you that citizens Andres Lopez and Miguel Venturas Arpeta were not kidnapped. They are currently serving their military service according to the law."

Later the families went to visit their two young men, Maria said. "And the family members came here then and told us, yes, they had seen them, the two of them. They were very worried about the two because they were doing forced labor. They were being given very little food. They were being forced to work the land without any tools, and so their hands were all wounded."

Under Guatemalan law, Maria said, the two men were ineligible for military service. One was too young, and the other was married and had a large family.

She took a deep breath. I began to think about other things I might have done with my time away from work—beaches I might have walked on, museums with beautiful art that I might have seen. But then the tears of the women in the next room came to mind, and I began to think of the two young soldiers who shouldn't be in the military. I thought, too, of Eliodoro Ordon Camey, and of his family.

Maria began to talk about assassinations. "Yesterday, the body of a university student appeared. The body was burned, tortured, and gunshot. So this is how we are living out the democracy that they say we are living in."

In a small way, I began to share in the sadness that permeated the GAM office, and I became aware of the resolution and strength of the people working there. I had felt strength and resolution in boardrooms, but they were of a different sort—a sort that comes from power wielded over time. In this room on the outskirts of Guatemala City, the strength and resolution I saw came not from power, but from pain endured over time.

Maria paused again and looked around the room. I realized that her expression had changed very little as she spoke.

A Kidnapped Brother

A member of our group broke the silence by saying, "I'd just like to relate that a friend of mine disappeared when I was in high school in the U.S. He was a youth leader in the high school." The man was Andrew Goodman, one of three young civil rights workers killed in Mississippi in 1964.

"So I just empathize, because in their case the whole country knew what happened, and the government took some kind of action. And here you're in a situation where the army *is* the Ku Klux

Klan, so to speak, and I just sympathize with the great difficulty you have and how much harder it is for you."

It was completely quiet again as Mary translated the man's comments to Maria Emilia Garcia, who listened with the same expressionless face that had characterized her recitation. She had been shaken by sorrow too often to react visibly, I decided. She nodded, and sitting close to her, I thought I saw the faint hint of a smile in her eyes. The man had touched her, I thought, and she was grateful for his comment.

"We are completely without help," she said simply.

I wondered what we in the United States would do if forty thousand people had been disappeared in Mississippi instead of just three.

"Is GAM able to speculate or figure out why these particular young men were singled out?" a member of our group asked.

Maria hesitated and looked over to the young man standing next to her as if to signal that he should respond.

"These men were peasant farmers," he said. "In the highlands, there's a lot of repression by the heads of the civil defense patrols and military commissioners. There's no doubt that they were being watched by the heads of their own patrols because they no longer wanted to participate in those patrols. So that was why they were persecuted."

Although the patrols are supposedly voluntary, not participating in them is a common cause of political violence in Guatemala. In practice, rural teenage boys and men of virtually every age and status are required to spend a full day each week monitoring activity in the immediate area, or working on roads for army vehicles. Something like ten percent of the population in Guatemala serves in the civil defense patrols.

Someone asked if the young man would tell us who he was. He laughed self-consciously and introduced himself as a member of GAM. He said he was an indigenous man from the department of El Quiche. But he did not give us his name.

There was pride in his voice when he said that he was indigenous, as though he wanted to be sure that we knew that he was still loyal to his culture, even though he was not dressed in traditional Indian clothing.

"I had a brother who was kidnapped," he said. "He was disappeared on December 5, 1981. At that time, we went to ask questions. We went to the military base. We looked in detention centers. But we were not able to find any information.

"Sometimes we went to look in the morgues and cemeteries, but we couldn't find him there either. My brother was not kidnapped alone, but with twenty-five other people. None of them have appeared. So that's why I'm involved with the group."

No Improvement

I asked if GAM ever got any help from the U.S. embassy, or from any particular church organizations. Several people snickered at the question, but Maria was patient, her composure unchanged. As happens so often, those who have been hurt are the most patient.

"From the U.S. embassy we've never received any help or support," she said. "And as far as church organizations, yes, we have received support. And from humanitarian groups in the United States as well as other parts of the world."

I expected her to elaborate on this, but she didn't, and someone asked if she would talk about what kind of action the government was taking against GAM members.

It was the young man who answered this question. He said, "In the interior of the country, members of GAM are being threatened if they continue to take part in our actions. They are accusing them of being guerrillas, because [the government says] GAM is the head of the guerrilla movement."

Someone else asked if there was any reason to expect the situation to improve. GAM had been hopeful when President Cerezo took office, Maria said. He had promised to investigate human rights abuses.

"But he defrauded us, because instead of helping us, what he did was approve the amnesty which gave protection to the military — those who we are accusing of the human rights violations. So we haven't been able to see any improvement. Exactly the opposite. Since the coup attempt of May 11, the situation has gotten worse.

"So, in the future, who knows how many years before the situation will improve. But the truth is we don't feel like we're on a road toward improvement."

Maria seemed tired. I have seen tired people in the business world—managers and employees who put in eighty hours a week for weeks at a time. But Maria's exhaustion ran deeper than theirs. It touched every part of her.

She said she had been working on the statistics for September. She was up to September 28. "There were sixty-eight assassinations, in addition to the disappearances, during that month."

There are fewer than nine million people in Guatemala. The rate of assassinations was running somewhere around one thousand per year. In the United States, that rate would yield about thirty thousand assassinations a year.

Still, the U.S. sends Guatemala almost two hundred million dollars in aid each year. Only eight countries in the world receive more foreign aid from the United States than Guatemala.

Even though this was only the second meeting of our trip, the first having been a briefing we received from Mary, I started to feel that something was terribly wrong in Guatemala, this tiny and violent country so close to our southern border.

Maria's monotone delivery and steady gaze, that same sad gaze we would see so often, spoke loudly without words the fact that the scars and the problems would remain for some time.

Clandestine Cemeteries

"What's happened with the clandestine cemeteries that they've discovered?" someone asked, referring to the rural gravesites that contain the bodies of many victims of the violence.

"That's been another demand and activity of the Mutual Support Group," Maria said, "that those clandestine graves be discovered, because there have been many denunciations that we've received here by family members who know where their loved ones are buried.

"But in order to be able to disinter their bodies, we need to go through a whole series of legal processes. And so the Mutual Support Group has gone through these legal procedures, but we've only been able to do that for two clandestine cemeteries. Both of them were in the department of El Quiche.

"In one, three bodies were found in one spot and two in another. They'd been assassinated in 1984, and the family members who were there recognized them in spite of the fact that there were just bones left. There was clothing that was still preserved.

"They could see the blood spots there. Their skulls had been split open as if by machete. And the bones, they could see, destroyed. And the relatives also recognized the two who were in the other grave."

In the second cemetery, Maria said, "Three were also found, three in one grave, and they were also recognized by their family members. They'd been killed in 1983, and these were also recognized because of the clothing."

As Maria described other attempts to recover bodies from clandestine cemeteries, I began to wonder what it would be like to know that the bodies of my loved ones were buried in a well near my household, or buried under rubble that couldn't be removed. I wondered what it would be like walking past the place, living nearby, remembering, not being able to unearth and honor the dead properly. Especially since, as Maria pointed out, "These people are religious and they want to give their family member a proper burial."

From a distance, it's difficult to feel another's pain. But I was close—a few feet away, across a dusty room. I tried to find a comfortable thought, a comfortable moment, a comfortable position on the hard floor, a comfortable topic to ease our minds, but there is little comfort to be found in Guatemala, except among the rich. And one must not be quick to condemn even the rich and powerful in Guatemala, because their comforts are superficial, and beneath these comforts they too have deep fears: fears for their security in this life, fears of their worth in the next.

Pontius Pilate

After another pause, during which she seemed to gather some energy, Maria talked about what GAM does beyond the denunciations and protests and attempts to recover the disappeared.

The relatives of the disappeared and other needy people come to the office every two weeks, she said. They're given corn, rice, beans, salt, oil, clothes, whatever GAM has. GAM tries to pay their bus fare if they come from far away. A medical clinic examines them, and provides prescriptions if they need them. The children are given vitamins, or treatment for worms or anemia. GAM members also work with the people on literacy when they can.

"It's difficult, but we're trying to move along little by little.

"On Father's Day, we take all these children so that the authorities can see how many children they have left without fathers," she said. "The children write messages or cards to their fathers. And we have a big board on which we put all of those messages."

I thought back to wonderful Father's Days with my family, and wanted us all to pause and say some kind of thanks for the privilege we had, a privilege that, until now, I had taken for granted.

But there was no such pause. A woman asked Maria if GAM ever solicited money from its supporters, by running ads for instance.

"No," Maria said. "We don't ask help in that way. It's too dangerous for those people."

Another woman asked about the government's human rights ombudsman. This time the young man answered. Maria clearly was getting tired. He said that a few months before, GAM had presented the ombudsman with information about kidnappings, including the names of the kidnappers. There had been no response.

"He always washes his hands by sending us to other institutions, and by saying that we have not provided enough information."

What Would She Ask?

A man asked if the Catholic Church had been supportive.

"The Catholic Church here really has not helped us," Maria said. "In the beginning, we went very frequently to the archbishop to ask if he would help us. But always what we received from him were words of consolation. He never took action to back up our demands.

"We've received telephone threats, sometimes anonymous written threats, papers thrown, defamation. But thanks to the international protection we have, things haven't gotten any worse than that."

Someone asked what we could do.

Maria thought for a moment, and without changing the pace or tone of her delivery she began in the middle of a thought. "Because not all North Americans are in human solidarity, we'd at least ask that those who are in solidarity be aware of what's going on in our country.

"And that you ask that our country not be armed so heavily in the tremendous way they're being armed. For example, recently we just got some arms that they said are the latest model. So they'll be replacing the ones that are no longer any good.

"They say that the guerrilla no longer exists here in Guatemala. And if the guerrilla no longer exists here, I don't know what they want those arms for, then. Because I think it was either today or yesterday that they said there are no longer guerrillas. And so if there's no one to fight, then why have the latest model weapons?

"And in terms of the GAM, we ask that you be aware of what's going on, and that you respond to whatever kind of call comes from us in whatever organization you belong to. And that you not forget also to send messages to the authorities here to demand that they respect the physical integrity of the members of the Mutual Support Group, reminding them that all of us have children and grandchildren that we have to protect. And there are many women who are alone, who earn their living by making tortillas in order to support their children."

With these last few words, Maria seemed to show that she was afraid. What I had seen up to now were her suffering and quiet determination. Now I thought about how fear could be buried deep inside, along with fatigue; I thought about how Maria's fear for herself was superceded by her fear for her loved ones and dependents.

It was time to stop, but we seemed reluctant to leave. We seemed to want to stay, and do something to help, some little thing, whatever it might be, maybe to make ourselves feel better, maybe to help ourselves forget.

I was afraid I was going to learn even more that I wouldn't like in our upcoming meetings in Guatemala, and I was right about that.

Pacaya

On the way out of the building, I took a copy of one of the GAM bulletins. It contained page after page of victims' names, followed by even more pages of newspaper stories about killings, disappearances, kidnappings, torture, and bodies that had been discovered.

That same day, one of the major local newspapers carried a large advertisement denouncing GAM as an organization led by women of loose morals, suggesting specifically that Nineth Montenegro de Garcia, Maria's daughter-in-law, was living in adultery and squandering GAM funds on personal pleasures. The ad was sponsored by the Fighters for Peace.

On March 25, 1989, the GAM offices were machine-gunned. On April 27, 1989, GAM discovered eight bodies in a clandestine cemetery located near Tunaja, Zacualpa, in El Quiche. GAM claimed that another hundred such cemeteries are still to be discovered in that district alone.

In August 1989, I learned that two members of Eliodoro Ordon Camey's family had been murdered since our visit.

During my work on this book, I learned that the volcano I saw so perfectly from the doorway of the GAM headquarters, Pacaya, had a special meaning for the Mutual Support Group. In the depths of its crater are the bodies of many of the disappeared.

Guatemala is a place where the political, economic, and social panorama is unfairly skewed in every possible way. In Guatemala, no one outside the charmed circle of the army and the very rich is safe, almost everyone is a victim in one way or another, and even those privileged few who remain immune from repression are conditioned by cowardice or greed.

Guatemala is a place where coups are plotted after minimal attempts at land reform, and where even talk of land redistribution is deemed "subversive" or communist. Guatemala is a place where those who have nothing offer the only chair in the house, while those who have everything will often not pay minimum wage. In Guatemala, life gets better for a minority, at the expense of millions of others.

In Guatemala, one doesn't have to carry a gun to be considered a "subversive." It is enough simply to want a better life for your children. Its citizens are abducted from downtown streets at midday before dozens of witnesses who dare not speak for fear of becoming victims themselves. Sometimes their tortured bodies are found, often unrecognizable. In the countryside, men are shot for carrying a dozen tortillas, since that much food in one man's hand must be destined for the "subversives," and those children who witness their parents' deaths grow up with a bitterness and resentment that will not ever be forgotten.

Jean-Marie Simon,
Guatemala: Eternal Spring, Eternal Tyranny
1987

The national security of all the Americas
is at stake in Central America.

If we cannot defend ourselves there,
we cannot expect to prevail elsewhere.

Our credibility would collapse,
our alliances would crumble,
and the safety of our homeland
would be put at jeopardy.

President Ronald Reagan
1983

2

Millionaire Bus Driver

Demographics

Guatemala is a beautiful country, roughly half the size of Minnesota. It is distinctly possible to visit it and never become aware of its suffering.

Within its forty-two thousand square miles, tourists can see over 750 species of orchids. Its scenic wonders include volcanoes, lakes, rivers, jungles, mountains rich with dark green foliage, and a great variety of animals and birds, one of which lends its name— *quetzal*—to the Guatemalan currency.

The country is a treasure chest for the archaeologist. At Tikal and elsewhere in the north, one can explore the ruins of the Mayan civilization, which thrived from 200 B.C. to almost A.D. 900, and made great strides in science, medicine, agriculture, astronomy, architecture, and mathematics. The Mayans developed both the concept of the zero and a solar calendar that is more accurate than the one we use today. The capital city of Guatemala is rich with museums offering evidence of the glories of past Central American civilizations.

For the tourist interested in modern cultures, a short trip to the highlands around Lake Atitlan, or to the Chichicastenango region, or even to the market of Guatemala City itself, offers the opportunity to study and enjoy Guatemala's rich ethnic mix, and the way that diversity manifests itself in language, dress, and customs. In the countryside, many Indians still wear their traditional costumes, and some still practice their ancient religions. Most still speak their own languages.

Guatemala is also a haven for the outdoor adventurer, who can find extraordinary whitewater river rafting, fishing, and deep-sea diving.

The country is rich in history as well. Materials abound to help one understand how the region fell to Captain Pedro de Alvarado in 1524, and how it lived under Spanish rule until independence came in 1821.

In four hours, an airplane can whisk the tourist from Chicago, New York, or Los Angeles to Guatemala City; from Miami, the trip takes two hours. In 1979, Guatemala welcomed some five hundred thousand tourists, but that number dropped steadily as the violence increased. In 1984, only two hundred thousand tourists came, but tourism has grown again under the Cerezo administration, and since the lifting of U.S. travel advisories.

U.S. economic aid to Guatemala has also increased, after having been suspended almost entirely during years of the most violent counterinsurgency campaign and human rights violations. In 1985, the Reagan administration began to supply Guatemala with considerable support; over $100 million was sent to the Cerezo government that year. In 1987, U.S. aid totaled $193 million.

The Guatemalan economy desperately needed aid. It was in a shambles following years of military struggle, inflation, growing foreign debt, population growth, political unrest, capital flight, and lack of investment due to the unstable environment.

Guatemala's foreign debt was just above $500 million in 1979. By 1985, it reached $2.5 billion, and it has grown since then. Soon it will reach a $3 billion level, or about half of the country's gross domestic product.

During the early 1980s, Guatemala's economy had a negative growth rate. In 1983 alone, the economy experienced an extraordinary drop of almost three percent. Economic growth in 1987 and 1988 was above two percent. Throughout the decade, however, the population grew by almost three percent each year.

Government spending is about ten percent of the gross domestic product—less than half the U.S. ratio. Agriculture accounts for one-fourth of the nation's economy, but provides two-thirds of its exports and sixty percent of its jobs. Wholesale and retail trade account for another one-fourth of the gross domestic product, manufacturing for sixteen percent, and the balance is taken up by a variety of utilities, banking, infrastructure, and private services.

In 1987, coffee exports exceeded $300 million, well over thirty percent of Guatemala's $1.1 billion export income. Bananas were the next largest export at $75 million, then sugar at $50 million, and cardamom at $45 million.

Much of the strength, or weakness, of the Guatemalan economy lies in the fortunes of its agricultural export industry.

Almost nine million people live in Guatemala, and the birth rate continues to be very high. There are almost forty births per thousand, against ten deaths, in spite of the poor living conditions of most Guatemalans.

A little less than half the population is Indian. The balance of the country is *ladino*. Most ladinos have mixed Spanish and Indian ancestry and are called *mestizos*; or they are Indians who, because of dress and lifestyle, are no longer identified with the culture of their ancestry.

Almost half the population now lives in urban areas, and Guatemala City feels the pressure of almost 3 million people, five times what its population was in 1974.

Another pressure building within Guatemala is the pressure of youth. Forty-seven percent of Guatemalans are under fourteen. Seventy-four percent are under thirty.

Unemployment figures are under fifteen percent, but they don't take into account the underemployed, and they don't consider the pressure building within this youthful population. Some estimates of unemployment are much higher.

A family needs almost nine quetzales a day to live with a proper, simple diet. Work in rural Guatemala, when it is available, pays less than half that amount.

The simple arithmetic of Guatemala's demographics is critical in assessing the country's future.

Development

FUNDESA was founded in 1984 by Guatemala's business elite to promote the country's economic health. The FUNDESA headquarters is in a high-rise office building in a new part of Guatemala City.

Security was tight when we entered the building. Heavily armed guards stood outside and monitored everyone's activities. We passed through a metal-detector gate like those in most airports, and once inside we were watched by still more armed guards.

On the building's top floor, however, we were treated to a magnificent view of Guatemala City. The exterior walls were glass, and the city spread out for miles in every direction. The slums were almost impossible to pick out from that height, and I found some sad poetry in that. Far more visible were the parks and playing fields, the other high-rise buildings, and the busy streets. I realized again how different things looked when you got far enough above them.

It was a sunny day with just a little breeze, and even the smog seemed thinner. In every way, I thought this visit would be a change of pace. In every way, that is, except for the guns of the security people downstairs.

We settled into one wing of the top floor, where chairs had been placed for us and a lectern with a microphone awaited our session. Our group leader introduced Maria Carmen Arsenia, the executive director of FUNDESA, and Carlos Chevas, the executive director designate, who would take Arsenia's place when her term ended. Then we were introduced to Juan Fernando Bendfelt, the director of studies and a member of the FUNDESA board of directors, who would speak with us.

"Basically I was asked to chat with you," Bendfelt said, "to maybe tell you what Guatemala is all about, and we chose this room rather than the standard meeting rooms below because this has the best view, and there it is." He gestured at the city spread out below us. "I have really very little to add.

"My point of view will be perhaps one, strictly, of an involved citizen and a businessman. How I see my country and the future.

"Let me tell you first a little bit about FUNDESA — the Guatemalan Development Foundation. It's a not-for-profit organization established by some twenty-five prominent businessmen in the community. Our task is to promote development. But as *we* understand development." He emphasized this last sentence.

"There has been a tremendous amount of mythology created in the last two decades around this word *development*. Half of the time when you think about development, you are probably associating it with projects funded by the Agency for International Development (AID), or with some type of subsidy or economic transfer."

FUNDESA had elected a different option, Bendfelt said. It promoted private investment to create both jobs and opportunities for foreign investment. It promoted legislation and conducted public relations efforts in support of its objectives.

"Our activities are basically trying to explain what the country is all about, trying to destroy some of these myths that for many years have created a very narrow point of view about what Guatemala is all about.

"So, in a way, we are constantly present, not only in the Guatemalan scenarios, but abroad. We try and reply to editorials that appear outside that are perhaps distorted or heavily biased or just outright lies that somebody has planted. Those are our activities."

FUNDESA produces a number of publications, he said. One is *Guatemala Watch*, a newsletter received by ten thousand readers in the United States each month. "Basically it's a collection of the most important news in the country.

"People are sometimes surprised when they come to the country, and they arrive to this modern metropolis with tall buildings and all this activity, which they were simply not even aware existed."

He said Guatemala City is the largest city in the Caribbean, with a population as large as the entire nation of Costa Rica.

"So there are a lot of things happening in the city that reflect urban lifestyles and are never portrayed abroad. We are a great deal more than a bunch of Mayans with a very poor economy. This is sometimes not evident to the foreign observer.

"And you will see that the presence of foreign names, like my own, is not a rarity. It's quite common. My family name dates to 1842, so that perhaps makes my family older than some of yours, as far as your family history coming from European immigrants. There are Guatemalans whose ancestors are German, a few British, and many Spanish.

"Nevertheless, the foreign community of Americans is also very prominent. We have an estimated population of U.S. visitors on the order of about ten thousand people, and these are not people related to a mission."

The number of U.S. citizens involved with charitable activities in Guatemala is large, he said. And a substantial number of Americans live in Guatemala.

"This dates back to the 1976 tragedy—the major earthquake that occurred at that time. After the earthquake, many of the organizations that came with aid and assistance for the emergency decided to undertake almost permanent projects. And so we do have a number of churches represented in Guatemala, with a number of important projects."

Religion

"FUNDESA and some of the other private-sector organizations have sponsored, for the past two or three years, some major public opinion surveys. We make a pretty comprehensive attempt to find out what the people think about a number of things."

Results of the most recent FUNDESA poll were prominently displayed in the October 1988 issue of *Guatemala Watch*, which we were given. Forty-three percent of those polled thought that President Cerezo was the fairest president in the country's history, and forty percent thought Cerezo was truly concerned about the poor. Sixty percent thought the May 1988 coup attempt had not been good for Guatemala. Twenty percent approved of the attempt. Over fifty percent thought Cerezo was creating a division between the rich and poor. Over sixty percent expected economic and social conditions to worsen in 1989. The method of polling was not described.

Bendfelt said almost thirty percent of all Guatemalans now identify themselves as non-Catholic Christians. "This, in terms of Latin America, is something which is perhaps unprecedented. It seems to many people like a very large amount.

"It has created some conflicts, since the Catholic Church does remain a major opinion force in the country, and that does explain some of the touchy areas in the relations of the church and the state at the moment."

Shifting gears suddenly, he said, "If you are still here and you don't have an anchor organization in Guatemala—a place where you can make probably a number of contacts—where we gather every Sunday is the Union Church of Guatemala.

"The Union Church many, many years ago was the only English-speaking Protestant church in the country. Now it's one of thousands, except that this is the place where most of the religious leaders gather. And they spend the rest of the week in their regular communities. People come from the countryside, and I invite you to come. Services are at eleven o'clock. Usually there's a coffee hour afterwards."

Three Basic Problems

Bendfelt went on, changing subjects rapidly and speaking in a businesslike drone. He had prepared a script, and he was going through it. He said Guatemala had been economically unique for a long time. Until 1980, it had a stable currency. In fact, it was so stable that the International Monetary Fund used it as a reference currency. The quetzal was pegged to the dollar.

"Obviously, after Mr. Carter's two-digit inflation, that created a crisis, because we were importing inflation by maintaining that fixed parity.

"Nevertheless, after the 1979 second oil crisis—and the spend-thrift Guatemalan government which created a budget deficit of nearly forty-eight percent of the actual expenditures—that stability was simply destroyed."

The Guatemala Central Bank tried to support an inflated purchasing power for the quetzal for a time in the early 1980s, Bendfelt said, and that strategy destroyed a second long-standing characteristic of the Guatemalan economy. Traditionally, Guatemala had a low foreign debt, especially in per capita terms. Now, Guatemala's foreign debt is a major concern.

"In the last five years, we have not experienced the kind of crisis the other Latin American countries experienced. We never had thousands of percent inflation per year. We never had 200, 300, 500 percent annual devaluations. And we did not have this tremendous tax burden.

"Between 1980 and today, we have had three major tax reforms, and a consistent attempt to almost double the size and the cost of government.

"Obviously, this was very much in vogue, even in the United States, in the late '30s and the '40s, and also in Argentina with Peron, and elsewhere. Somehow Guatemala was excluded from this world trend, and this accounted for Guatemalan prosperity and stability for many, many years.

"This is not the case anymore. And as a result of that, we are experiencing a recurrent and constant number of tensions—political tensions, social tensions—derived from this adjustment.

"It is something that the private sector has not supported, the growth of government.

"Nevertheless, I have to admit that it has been your government—State Department, AID—that has consistently supported this view, that Guatemalans need to pay more taxes and the Guatemalan government needs to get involved in more and bigger things.

"And also, by providing foreign assistance in near-free conditions, the foreign debt keeps growing. This, we believe firmly, is not the path to prosperity, but is simply the path to put Guatemala in the same place where everybody else in Latin America is.

"At a time when some other countries are trying to look like Guatemala looked like a few years ago, we are sort of borrowing a trend which is no longer viewed as a road to prosperity around the world."

Bendfelt stopped. We, his audience, sat stoically. After hearing about widows and orphans, about violence and human rights, this discussion about foreign debt, currency fluctuations, and whether large or small government was the key to prosperity struck me as flat and unfeeling.

Culture

Bendfelt may have sensed the flatness of our response; in any case, he moved to a subject that touched me more closely.

Guatemala, he said, from the time of its conquest, was different from "Mexico, the Caribbean, or even in the United States, where basically the indigenous population was either wiped out or removed or simply discarded into the boondocks."

At the time of the conquest, he said, the population of Central America was concentrated in Guatemala. Elsewhere the population was scattered and sparse. Guatemala City is one of the oldest cities in the world if one traces back beyond the Spanish conquest.

"One of the oldest archaeological sites in Guatemala City is called Kaminal Juyu, and Kaminal Juyu dates back several thousands of years before Christ, and this valley has been populated constantly since then."

Guatemala was conquered by a handful of Spanish soldiers, he said—perhaps twenty, "some ridiculous number." But they recruited an army of Mexican Indians, and they had horses, and these two things made the difference.

The Spanish then faced the problem of how to rule with just a few Spaniards and an army of mercenaries. They decided they had no choice but to preserve the culture—or cultures, since over twenty Indian tribes lived in Guatemala, each with its own language. These tribes were unrelated to the original Mayans.

The major Mayan sites, such as Tikal, had been abandoned by the eleventh century. After that, waves of Mexican tribes immigrated into the area. "By the time the Spanish conquerors came, the Indian culture was already pretty decadent," he said, meaning that it could no longer sustain the glories the Mayan civilization had achieved.

"When the Spanish came, we find these splintered groups warring against each other."

Today, four major languages are spoken by the Guatemalan Indians—Quiche, Cakchiquel, Mam, and Kekchi.

"The point, in fact, is that when you look at one of these Indian Guatemalans, they deserve more respect than we actually pay them," he said. "Many of them speak more than three languages, which is something that very few other Guatemalans can claim."

They have the language of their tribe. If it is what Bendfelt called a secondary tribe, they must learn one of the four major Indian languages. They often learn Spanish, and in some of the tourist areas, they learn English as well.

"So a great number of them speak up to four languages, which is something that is always overlooked when you evaluate this culture."

The survival of the languages, Bendfelt said, indicates that the Spanish preserved the indigenous cultures, and understanding that cultural heritage is important, because seventy percent of the population is of Indian descent.

I would learn later that some people feel Bendfelt gave credit where it wasn't due by suggesting the Spanish preserved the indigenous cultures.

"But we have fundamentally two cultures," he said. "What we would call the Western-oriented, urban culture of Guatemala City, and then the traditional Indian culture. There is a particular anthropological definition that Guatemalans have created to describe this process of changing from the Mayan traditional culture to the urban, Occidental way of life. We call those people ladinos."

Then Bendfelt said proudly that Guatemala "has no restrictions of any kind, legally or even culturally, on this process of merging." Many prominent Guatemalans, he said, have Indian ancestry — even the president of FUNDESA.

"Some of the major problems in the countryside, in the little towns, arise not between what we would call the creole, or mestizos, who have some European blood, but arise between these two Indian cultures: one that's very conservative — the self-preserving culture — and the one that has left its culture to move into Western society."

The cultural conflict within the Indian communities accounts for the conflict among the churches as well, Bendfelt said. The Catholic Church maintains a strong presence within the traditional Indian society, whereas among the ladinos "you have this flourishing, booming growth of the Christian [fundamentalist] churches."

Cultural Change

Because of this ethnic and cultural mix, Bendfelt said, change is very difficult. "A foreigner, or even somebody from the city, cannot go out there and promote change, even if change means some good things, like water and drainage and communications.

"It's a society dominated by men, and dominated still by these traditional families, sort of like the Cabots and Lodges in Boston were thirty, forty, fifty years ago. Everybody else doesn't count. That is still pretty much the description of what an Indian community in this traditional culture experiences."

We found on our trip, however, that women are emerging everywhere as active participants and leaders. Moreover, the remaining dominance of men seemed to be as present in other segments of Guatemalan society as it was in the Indian communities.

Among the women, he said, there is a low level of literacy. The men are the ones who go to school, learning some basic skills — reading, writing, a little accounting, before they leave school.

"Just as a word of warning, consider the fact that trying to change these people would also put in danger their traditional ways of life. And this is something which is very seldom valued when policy is being directed by somebody from AID, or somebody simply looking at the statistics."

It is commonly suggested, Bendfelt said, that Guatemalans need to be educated, but the uneducated would resist. They would expect to be taught absurd things, things they don't need and don't want. So there is tremendous tension between those who want change and those who do not.

Guatemala's military-dominated government allowed the development of a new constitution in 1985. Parts of it were beneficial, Bendfelt said. Before that, the government "was conceived of as a single cash register, and as a single checkbook. So you can understand that the two most powerful people in the government, and in the country, were related to the Ministry of Finance in the government of Guatemala."

He said nothing about the matter of amnesty for past human rights violations.

The new constitution requires eight percent of the national budget to be disbursed directly to the individual communities "for them to throw away, or spend, or invest, or use as they so desire," Bendfelt said. He urged us to look carefully as we toured the country, to notice the changes resulting from these direct disbursements.

We did look carefully, and saw only one sign of the use of such funding which happened to be a road repair project that some people thought benefited the military more than the peasants. Later I would learn that there is substantial doubt about whether the eight percent actually gets disbursed the way the constitution intended.

"Maybe they are introducing water; maybe they're paving their streets; maybe they're putting a kiosk in their central park, or rebuilding their church, or whatever. I think this is really one of the few very positive things that has come out of the new constitution."

He said the Christian Democrats were trying to take all the credit for this generosity, rather than saying that it was the result of the constitution. Still, Bendfelt said, the impact would be good. Democracy would take on real meaning, because now there would be money involved.

"They will have to discover some kind of system by which they will arrive at decisions," he said. "And, of course, democracy is the best system." He said there was no tangible reason to push for democracy before the constitutional change, but that now there was.

In many Indian communities, however, he said the real power lay not with the political organizations and officials, but with the traditional Indian hierarchy.

"If you are going to Lake Atitlan, it is amazing what you can find in this, which is the smallest department in the country. It has perhaps the greatest cultural diversity. You have three of the major tribes dividing the lake, and even among the Quiche, who are the most numerous, you have some tremendous differences from one community to the next."

In Solola, on the north shore of Lake Atitlan, the elders of the Indian tribe change at the end of the year. "They are the real power," he said. "And any day that you go to the town, you will realize that there is a line of people just waiting for these elders to pass judgment on their issues and their conflicts. They are still operating pretty much in their ancient tribal ways, and the system has worked."

In summary, Bendfelt said Guatemala was probably a confusing place for us. "I would simply ask you to put your prejudices aside, and then try to look beyond what is apparent, particularly before you pass judgment on their culture, and our culture, which is, I think, emerging from this melting pot, which is really not destroying the ancient ways, but simply accommodating them."

Carter's Blunders

A group member asked if Bendfelt expected any change in U.S. policy under President Bush. He said no, he didn't, and he was sorry that was the case. He had hoped for change when President Reagan came into office.

"Mr. Carter made three serious blunders that we are paying a great deal more for than you are, although you are paying the bill."

The first mistake, he said, was the Panama Canal treaty, which had the effect of shifting the power structure in Central America.

"Second was giving away Nicaragua to the Marxist regime. It was a unilateral handout, done by the State Department, against all the Organization of American States agreements." During the last day before the fall of Managua, he said, the U.S. ambassador supplied weapons to the Sandinistas rather than the National Guard, and this was well documented.

The third error had to do with El Salvador. The U.S. began pushing for reform, undemocratically, during the time of the junta, which followed the coup overthrowing General Romero. During this time, banks were nationalized, agricultural exports were nationalized, and agrarian reform programs were put into place, he said, and these three things destroyed the private property system of El Salvador.

"Now this is all created at the time of Mr. Carter. We all hoped that Mr. Reagan would come into office with a, let's say, clear vision of these three mistakes. Instead of that, for eight years, the situation has been stalling. And for the last three years, the Central Americans are in a process of accommodation to this reality, which we think is here to stay."

Regional Outlook

"First of all, the Sandinistas will remain there," Bendfelt said. "Even if they come to some kind of an agreement to stop sending arms to the Guatemalan and Salvadoran guerrillas, and stop the training of guerrillas for the eventual insurgency in Costa Rica and Honduras. This is well documented.

"As has happened throughout the world, as soon as they are again prepared to confront a weaker U.S. government, they will reinitiate this."

He described Guatemalan foreign policy as "active neutrality." Guatemala wants the Nicaraguans to resolve their internal issues by themselves. Yet, he said, Guatemala favors democracy and continuing dialogue to promote peace.

As he spoke, I realized that although he showed little feeling, he seemed to be enjoying himself. He moved easily through facts, ideas, and words that landed almost without emotional impact on him or his audience.

He went on at a steady pace, noting that Guatemala had opposed the Reagan initiatives designed to remove the Sandinistas from power, and that had prevented a united Central American position on Nicaragua. "Consistently, President Cerezo and his advisors have undermined the firm position of the United States. But once we have these Sandinistas in confinement, there will be this ever-present danger of them simply exporting their product, which is terrorism."

A year later, while finishing this book, I realized that terrorism is always what the other guy does. By definition, the good guys are defenders and the bad guys are terrorists. Bendfelt never mentioned death squads, disappearances, or a military trained in torture techniques and psychological warfare, all things deliberately designed to terrorize anyone who might rebel, denounce, protest, or seek reform.

Bendfelt predicted change in El Salvador. "The Salvadoran electorate has spoken. They are tired of the Christian Democrats, and it was a landslide. If the ARENA party comes to power, there probably will be a resurgence of the military conflict, with the support of the population."

One expert told me later that the landslide Bendfelt claimed for ARENA was actually earned with the votes of less than twenty percent of those who were eligible.

Bendfelt cautioned us not to believe everything we read about El Salvador, and especially about the ARENA party. He said the press often connected ARENA with death squads and with the murder of Archbishop Romero, and that the connections might not be appropriate.

Regarding El Salvador, "The conflict now is designed by sociologists, defined as a low-intensity conflict, designed to allow them to maintain some positions but not really bring an end to the conflict."

As far as the Guatemalan guerrillas were concerned, he thought they no longer received as much support as they had from outside the country, and that this was "part of the deal by which Guatemalan foreign policy took the shape of neutralism." As a result, the number of guerrilla initiatives was lower, especially near the Mexican border.

"Again, this has some good points, but also some bad points. Not all of the four guerrilla groups in Guatemala are very obedient to the directions that come from Managua and Cuba. They are pretty much independent Marxists." The fear now was that the guerrillas would move into the cities and increase the level of urban terrorism.

Millionaire Bus Drivers

A man asked Bendfelt to speak to the skewed distribution of wealth in Guatemala. For the first time, I thought Bendfelt was no longer enjoying himself. He reacted angrily to the question.

"Do you know which country in the world has the most unequal distribution of land?" He let the question hang in the air until everyone had guessed the answer. "It's the United States." Then he tempered his attack by explaining that the disparity in Guatemalan land ownership was not important.

"There is no connection whatsoever between this idea of land distribution patterns and prosperity," he said. In fact, he claimed, prosperous economies had fewer people involved in the production of food.

The questioner wasn't satisfied. He said the inequity went beyond the question of land, and involved all the wealth of the country.

Bendfelt asked how long we had been in the country. When he learned it had been only a few days, he smiled.

He told us a story about a man who attended the constitutional convention in 1985. The man was illiterate in Spanish. People thought it was awful that such a man was involved in this important process, until they found out more about him.

"The man was a self-made millionaire," Bendfelt said.

"He was the largest private bank, himself, in that area. He had forty buses, and each one of these buses cost something like twelve thousand dollars. And there was an interview in the press that told his story, how he became this banker and transportation millionaire.

"Big business, big business," Bendfelt exclaimed in one of his more animated moments. He said the man started as a peon on the coffee farms, "which is pretty much what many of the people in the highlands do to complement their food production with hard cash. That's how he started. Nevertheless, if you met this millionaire in the street, you would never, never know who you were talking to."

When the man bought his first bus, Bendfelt said, he entered the dealership with his money in his satchel. He wore no shoes. He couldn't speak Spanish. The sales people were going to throw him out. He had to show them his cash just to get their attention.

"This is the type of thing that is not evident," Bendfelt said. "Just because they are Indians, and they look poor, don't think they are. The statistics don't tell half the truth."

Distortions

A woman asked about the foreign press, which Bendfelt had said sometimes distorted things about Guatemala, and whether he would expand on that comment. Bendfelt pointed to the statistics on the distribution of wealth as an example of distortion. "This is something that is constantly mentioned whenever there's a reference to Guatemala."

This questioner, however, like the last one, was persistent and wanted to know what would motivate people to misrepresent Guatemala.

People are prejudiced, Bendfelt said, getting angry again. They want to change things. "Especially the liberal media of the United States, which is infiltrated with this.

"I know more about what's happening in the world by reading a Guatemalan newspaper than by reading any newspaper in the world, aside from the five major ones in the United States. You will find Mrs. Jones's cat had an accident, or somebody got married, or a funeral, but as far as news, there is hardly any news."

But what was the motivation to distort? the woman asked. Well, Bendfelt said, it was their political "mission," their vision of how society should be. There again, if you want to promote change in the area, analyze what the cost would be. The costs in many respects mean destroying this ancient culture.

"Many of the problems that come from abroad come with this idea—they want to produce change. As a result, there is conflict, or rejection. Preachers get kicked out of towns."

He was interrupted by the man who had asked about the unequal distribution of income, who said he needed a clarification. Did Bendfelt mean that the statistics are right but just weren't interpreted accurately?

"Yes," Bendfelt said. "You weren't being consistent with that idea, that there's something wrong because there's this concentration of land. The most likely place in the world where agrarian reform should distribute land to everybody is the United States. Now, I have yet to hear any of you, or any American, propose that."

The meeting was starting to deteriorate. Most of the group seemed hostile to Bendfelt's end of the political spectrum to begin with, and his answers and tone were exacerbating that hostility. I wondered if Bendfelt wouldn't preemptively end the session soon.

Bendfelt recovered his poise quickly, however. He seemed to enjoy the give and take, but I doubted he had much respect for us.

He said the land in Guatemala was very productive. As land became more productive, ownership tended to concentrate into fewer hands. It was a normal, desirable process.

The group was skeptical, and Bendfelt returned to his bus driver.

"It's not one of these rare cases. If you go to the bus terminal of Guatemala City, or if you look at any of the buses that are constantly moving in the countryside, look at the driver. Ninety-five percent of the time the driver is the owner. Then you will realize that these people, they are Indian or of Indian background."

I was surprised, or rather, amazed, that Bendfelt refused to leave the illustration of the bus owners; it seemed clear that his credibility was nonexistent on this point, and that hurt his credibility on everything else he said.

A voice inside me, however, said not to be too harsh in judging this man. In many ways, I identified more with him than with the people at GAM; it was simply a matter of where we spent most of our time—in the business world, where the primary emphasis is on making money.

Bendfelt said the statistics were also heavily distorted simply because Guatemala had a large nonmonetary economy. "The small peasant farmer tills his land, produces his harvest. That harvest is never accounted for in the statistics. He simply puts it in his warehouse and then uses it."

We had just spent a week traveling in Honduras, where I saw no rural warehouses. I made a mental note to look carefully for such warehouses in Guatemala. I never saw any.

"So the income statistics don't register. The per capita income statistics in Guatemala are horrendously distorted. We don't know by how much." He said FUNDESA was trying to promote research to get at the correct data.

"It's an outright lie when the World Bank comes and tells us, 'Whoops, you're one of the poorest countries in the world, with an annual per capita income of a hundred dollars.' We think that's not congruent with what we see in reality."

A young man asked where we might be able to help. Bendfelt said that if we weren't willing to invest and create jobs, "If you just want to help somebody financially, go to the very needy. The *very* needy.

"In particular, in the case of Guatemala, we're experiencing something which is, just like you have the baby boomers, we could have a similar type of shock with the more than a hundred thousand orphans from the earthquake."

The room was silent. I knew about Guatemala's orphans, and about the earthquake that killed over twenty thousand people in a brief, horrible moment. But Bendfelt lost further credibility with me by refusing to add that the orphans were also a result of the political violence in Guatemala, which has intensified during the past decade. No one followed up on the issue.

Caribbean Basin Initiative

A man asked about the Caribbean Basin Initiative — called CBI.

"We think it's a wonderful idea," Bendfelt said. "I am very much in favor of free trade and low tariffs. This works both ways. It benefits the U.S. consumers with better prices, and it also benefits our area with investments and jobs.

"It has created this export-oriented mentality in the local business community which will eventually identify many other opportunities than those provided by CBI. It has created self-confidence and self-esteem."

Nontraditional exports were increasing, he said — fresh crops, for example.

There was a catch, however. Most of the things Guatemala could export were exempt from the CBI. "So the actual economic benefit is very small." And there were other problems. Freight rates were terrible. Products could be imported from the Far East at low rates, but from Guatemala to Miami the rates were very high, perhaps six times as high.

"Why? Because in the case of Guatemala, all of the transportation and communications systems are still owned by the government. They are not only very inefficient — they hardly even work — but they are also very expensive. To protect the national airline, air fares to Guatemala have consistently been higher per mile than anywhere else.

"So, I think that the idea of privatizing the state-owned enterprises, and deregulation, should go hand in hand with promoting exports.

"The telephone system, for example. I don't know if any of you have tried to call home, but good luck."

He was interrupted by laughter. Many of us had been frustrated in our attempts to place long-distance calls.

He said he could only get through early in the morning or during lunch. Anyone who had to keep in continual touch with world markets was in trouble simply because of the telephone system.

"So that explains a little bit why we haven't jumped aggressively, because the infrastructure is all state controlled."

Guatemalan Universities

The priest in our group asked him to comment on Guatemala's university system.

"San Carlos University is one of the oldest," Bendfelt said. "It's the third oldest university in Latin America. But it became the haven of Marxists."

About twenty-five years ago, he said, other private universities were able to obtain charters. Now there were five such schools. San Carlos was still the largest, with almost fifty thousand students. A Catholic school had about eight thousand. Marroquin University had about six thousand. The other two colleges were smaller.

One difficulty facing higher education was simply that there weren't enough jobs. The graduates had few opportunities to put their skills to use.

Bendfelt was especially critical of the quality of agricultural education at San Carlos.

"They are more concerned with educating economists, humanists, lawyers. So there is very little connection between what the market is demanding and the orientation of the state university. This is not the case with the other schools."

He was, he said, a trustee at one of those other schools. Not surprisingly, he felt that his school was quite successful. Before they set their curriculum, they had studied what was happening at the other schools.

"After analyzing that the academic community, the university professors, scientists, literary figures, all these intellectuals were actually debasing the foundations of the free society of Guatemala, what the University of Marroquin set out to do was to straighten out that record."

They decided to educate economists and lawyers, exactly what the other universities were turning out. But, the Marroquin economists and lawyers are trained with a different philosophy, he said.

"As a result of that, we began our program, and we are now seventeen years old. You will find our graduates placed in key positions of leadership in the business community, and changing the economy of the country. We are a free-market oriented university. But our vision, which is very much one-sided, is not shared by everyone else."

A man asked him to comment further on the university situation and what might be needed to effect improvements.

One problem, Bendfelt said, was that it was too easy for students to attend San Carlos. Three percent of the country's budget went to support San Carlos, and no questions were ever asked about how the money was spent. He called the situation "a horrendous privilege." It was too easy to be admitted, and too inexpensive for the students. "Few ever graduate," he said.

"But this is a very touchy issue, particularly when you find that the Marxist intellectuals from the university have connections with the guerrilla movement. Many suspect that this legal haven is used for very illegal subversive activities in general."

Power Structure

Someone asked him to describe the power structure in Guatemala.

"Well the power structure in Guatemala changes." At election time, the power shifted to the political parties, he said. But after the elections people joined the winning party as a way to keep their jobs.

Bendfelt said the political parties were not strong enough to shape the country's political and social agenda. The true power rested with the ruling party, which controlled the lawmaking. Laws they wanted were passed easily. Other laws lingered endlessly. The Christian Democrats dominated both the presidency and the congress.

Bendfelt didn't mention it, but Guatemalan president Cerezo is on record claiming he possesses only twenty percent of the power his office is supposed to have.

The situation was not democratic, Bendfelt said. Opposition voices could not be heard. Opposition initiatives, such as the denationalization of industry, or the export incentives FUNDESA would like, were ignored.

The Catholic Church was still very powerful, Bendfelt said. The Church used to be "a state-sponsored institution." It enjoyed almost equal power with the state until independence, in the early nineteenth century. After losing that, however, it still enjoyed tremendous power.

The Church's situation was changing, though. "The Catholic Church is experiencing changes that are perhaps not for the better. For many years, the prior archbishop [Cardinal Mario Casarriego], who was very conservative, kept a very close rein on his organization. Right now, that is not the case.

"And we have a tremendous number of European priests who have come, and there have been Canadian religious women's organizations that are very active in this country. Many of them share this vision of Liberation Theology."

He said the Catholic Church is now calling for agrarian reform.

A third major force was the military, he said. Constitutional requirements now provided for retirement and rotation, making a coup more difficult to engineer.

"The laws require at least twenty-seven positions of command. There is a continuous rotation. It's a very professional standing army, and people are forced into retirement once they are out of commission or they have reached a number of years of service. So maybe this has brought better control of the army. But still, it's a very powerful political force."

Finally, the private sector was very strong, he said. He made a point of distinguishing between the private sector and the oligarchy. He had no desire to communicate that power was concentrated in the hands of a few.

"There are numerous organizations. You will also see that the system is not closed to the small, the medium businessman. It's a very open system; a very open system."

Topics Not Mentioned

It was time to stop. Our hosts had filled tables with coffee and soft drinks.

Before we adjourned, the priest in our group thanked Bendfelt for his perspective and his candor. We gave Bendfelt a polite round of applause, but, atypically, few of us went up to the podium for a private question or conversation.

I felt that a good deal of what Bendfelt said was worth careful consideration. Still, I didn't feel comfortable with him, especially compared to the people I'd met the day before. They were struggling for something. In many ways, their situation wasn't as complex or as distant. It was true that Bendfelt had forced us to see some parallels between Guatemala and the United States. He had shown us that the situation was complex, especially given the country's cultural and ethnic traditions, and the region's political turmoil.

But he was untouched, above it all in this tenth-floor room. The suffering was out of sight. He never talked about starvation, or illiteracy, or unemployment, or slums, and no one asked him to do so. He never mentioned corruption, violence, assassinations, or the disappeared. The orphans he wanted us to think about were the ones orphaned by the earthquake.

I could appreciate Bendfelt's intellect, but I couldn't feel much softness in his heart. Why would he meet with us at all, I wondered. Perhaps to tell us that we had problems too; that we were part of the problem in Guatemala; that we should mind our own business; that, with all its problems and complexity, Guatemala was doing a good job, maybe even a decent and caring job; that the Christian Democratic Party was too socialist and San Carlos University too Marxist.

He was a confident man, and I wondered where that confidence came from. Having listened to Maria Emilia Garcia and Juan Fernando Bendfelt, I wasn't at all confident that I could put the pieces together.

Bendfelt brought me back to the reality of ideological struggle—laissez-faire capitalism versus socialism, the private sector versus the public sector, and what some people call East versus West. I thought the word fascism fit in there somewhere, too.

Still, my sense was that the larger struggle had to do with the simple realities of wealth and power—true democracy versus disenfranchisement; a few people with more than enough versus many with too little; the haves versus the have-nots.

However this *ladino* minority thinks its blood is superior,
a higher quality,
and they think of Indians as a sort of animal.
That's the mark of discrimination.

The *ladinos* try to tear off this shell which imprisons them
—being the children of Indians and Spaniards.
They want to be something different,
they don't want to be a mixture . . .

At the same time there are differences between *ladinos* too;
between rich *ladinos* and poor *ladinos*.
The poor are considered lazy,
people who don't work,
who only sleep and who have no enjoyment in life.

But between these poor *ladinos* and Indians
there is still that big barrier.
No matter how bad their conditions are,
they feel *ladino*,
and being *ladino* is something important in itself:
it's not being an Indian.

I, Rigoberta Menchu
1984

Then the righteous will answer him,
"Lord, when did we see thee hungry and feed thee,
or thirsty and give thee drink?
And when did we see thee a stranger and welcome thee,
or naked and clothe thee?
And when did we see thee sick or in prison and visit thee?"

And the King will answer them,
"Truly, I say to you,
as you did it to one of the least of these my brethren,
you did it to me."

Matthew 25:34–40

3

Poorest of the Poor

Forbidden Things

On Wednesday morning, November 23, 1988, we met in an outer room next to a church in Guatemala City with a priest who was active in several social initiatives. To give his name or say much about what he does would endanger him. Although he is now in exile outside Guatemala after receiving one too many death threats, he is not out of danger and does hope to return. I'll call him Padre Tomas.

Padre Tomas was a thin man, perhaps in his forties. Like Maria Garcia, he spoke calmly and steadily. He had worked in Central America, and especially Guatemala, for several decades.

"I understand that you have an interest in the role that the United States plays here, and an interest in the churches in Guatemala. I'll give a short talk about these things, and then I'll open up for any questions you might have.

"Both the Catholic and Protestant churches suffered repression in these last years in a terrible way. In only one of our parishes, we have twenty thousand widows, and the majority of those women had husbands who were working with the Church.

"When President Rios Montt came into power [in 1982], the Church felt great relief that maybe the persecution would end, because the anguish and the violence were so terrible. But that didn't happen. The repression continued very violently.

"As in the rest of Central America, but probably in a worse way, the union of the army and the private sector are what control

the country. And having this new civilian come to the head of the
government—" He paused and shook his head to indicate that
President Cerezo made no difference whatsoever.

"Now we have a new civil government, a new face, but the
people who still run this country are, in fact, the military.

"When the Church tries to talk about things that are very deep
and necessary, such as human rights, such as land ownership, these
are forbidden things. You can tell that there's been an agreement
between Cerezo and the military that these subjects will not be
touched.

"This helps you understand why the pastoral letter of the
bishops, 'The Cry for Land,' has been criticized very, very severely,
publicly, in the newspapers. No other hierarchy in any part of the
world has received such criticism. They are accused of being ignorant, of playing up to communism, to disqualify the entire
letter."

"The Cry for Land"

"The Cry for Land," the extraordinary pastoral letter of the
Guatemalan bishops on land reform, argues that land ownership
has not only been a serious problem for Guatemala for a long time,
but that in recent years the problem has become more severe.

Guatemalan land ownership is concentrated in the hands of the
very few. In 1979, two percent of the farms held two-thirds of the
land. One percent of the farms represented twenty percent of the
land. At the other extreme, ninety percent of the farms had just over
fifteen percent of the land. Since then, the skew has become worse.
Bendfelt's assertion that this distortion isn't significant stood in
stark contrast to the bishops' data.

"There are many problems afflicting our brothers and sisters in
the rural areas in their long calvary of suffering," the bishops write.
"However, their dispossession of the land should be considered the
nucleus of the social problem in Guatemala.

"It is a fact that the majority of arable land is in the hands of a
privileged few, while the majority of peasants own no plot of land

on which to sow their crops. This situation, far from pointing toward a solution, becomes day by day more harsh and painful.

"Certainly the critical problem of land ownership is at the very heart of the propagation of injustice."

Of the peasants' desire for land, the bishops say, "Theirs is a legitimate cry."

They repeat the words of Pope John Paul II in his homily in Guatemala in 1983: "To forestall any extremism and to consolidate an authentic peace, there is no better way than to return their dignity to those who suffer injustice, contempt and misery."

There is no plea for socialism in the "The Cry for Land." The right of private property is acknowledged and accepted. But the bishops qualify the right of private property; they impose limitations. They quote John Paul II on the subject: "The earth is a gift from God, a gift God makes to every human being, men and women, whom God wants gathered together in a single family and related to one another with a spirit of friendship. It is not right, therefore, because it is not in harmony with God's plan, to use this gift in such a way that the earth's benefits favor just a few, leaving others, the immense majority, excluded. . . . Nothing we have spoken of can come about unless we accept the idea that a change of sinful and obsolete social structures is necessary and urgent in Guatemala," the bishops state.

Land Ownership and Refugees

Padre Tomas continued. "Today the bishops, in their bishops' conference, have become the belligerent ones. Eight years ago we, as clergy, were criticized by the bishops for our belligerence, and today it's the bishops who are being accused of being communists. So now we feel that our work here is much more united. So, for the first time we feel we are able to support what our bishops are doing."

Padre Tomas didn't speculate about the reasons for the change. Instead, he changed the subject abruptly.

"The civil patrols in the interior, the military commissioners, they are the very well-organized control that we have in our coun-

try. The disappearances still continue, and there's an endless number of assassinations. And there's been pressure on pastoral agents
in different parts of the country.

"In El Quiche, they have forbidden the entrance of a Jesuit
priest. They have pressured another priest to leave El Quiche. And
the catechists still do not have the confidence that they had before
the severe pressure came."

Catechists had been one of the primary targets of the political
violence, and were still carefully watched by the military and its
spies.

"Two things, I think, are great problems, social as well as political: ownership of the land, and the refugees — one of the most deli-
cate themes that needs to come up in the national dialogue."

Over one million people have been displaced by the violence of
recent years. The refugees are those people still unsettled.

Refugees are often considered the equivalent of guerrillas by
the Guatemalan power structure. Because of that, refugees have little voice in the national dialogue, a process resulting from the Central American Peace Accords. The dialogue is supposed to be a forum to resolve differences and solve problems peacefully.

"The government is disputing the legality of the refugees,
which would make them unable to join the discussion," Padre Tomas said. "GAM — those women and men who represent all the disappeared of Guatemala — they're also kept out of the dialogue as
communists or guerrillas, or whatever.

"And so any group like that that wants to speak about land
ownership or human rights, they are pushed over to one side and
they are trying to eliminate them from that conversation."

Democracy and Elections

"Now, let's talk about the United States," Padre Tomas said.
"Guatemala can be seen in a different light with respect to the United States than the rest of Central America. The military here has always been very nationalistic, and at various times they have reject-
ed U.S. policies.

"And that's probably the only way they're different, because like the other armies in Central America, they have a great deal of power and control.

"We think the line that the government and the army use has been provided for them by the United States. It's called 'democratized society, Central America.' And when we talk about democracy, that means democracy U.S. style.

"Because of Nicaragua, they are insisting on a democracy that comes out of elections, and not a democracy that comes out of participation by the whole country. If there are elections, that's sufficient."

I had never accepted without reservation the idea that the use of ballot boxes means that democracy is alive and well. But only when I began studying Central America's recent history did I understand how little elections mean there. They have often been fraudulent. And, even when they are relatively honest, elections do not guarantee a sharing of power, or meaningful participation in the formulation of social policy and programs.

Returning to his comments about the United States, Padre Tomas said, "They don't pressure us about land ownership. They don't pressure us to include popular participation. They don't pressure for popular organization. And they give a free hand to the army."

Fundamentalist Sects

Without a pause, Padre Tomas began to list U.S. influences on Guatemala. The first thing he mentioned was the Pentagon. The second was the religious fundamentalists from the U.S.

"They have multiplied from two percent to twenty-four percent," he said. "They had their highest point at the time of Rios Montt. This curve has now gradually declined. In some dioceses we even have ceremonies to receive members back again."

President Rios Montt was a fundamentalist. His short term in office, during 1982 and 1983, marked the most violent years of Guatemala's history. The guerrilla movement, which seemed about to succeed, was driven back into hiding, and tens of thousands died.

"Some studies indicate that the greater the repression is, the more the fundamentalist sects abound. In some places, to be an evangelical means you're safe to live. For example, those refugees who are in Mexico, forty thousand countrymen. Those who can come back to Guatemala, they have come back under the Central American Church, which is a fundamentalist church, which we think was the church of Rios Montt some years ago.

"The most serious problem for us as believers are these Protestant sects, including some Catholic sects. Some charismatic groups can be called sects. [Their work results in] the division and destruction of the indigenous culture. There is no place for ecumenism. Those groups destroy the anthropological life and the culture of the people. I think that's the greatest problem that the sects have created.

"There are some good aspects in them. They fight against alcoholism. They struggle against breaking up families. They try to develop the person. We can applaud that, and see that's beneficial.

"But that is at the cost of destroying their culture. Everything is taken. Everything that belongs to their tradition is considered pagan and must be destroyed. And this will not be pardoned by the indigenous peoples in the future.

"And this strategy of North American missionaries who come from the churches has been part of United States strategy towards our country."

Padre Tomas ended his presentation and asked if we had questions.

A woman said, "I'd be interested to know some of the things the Church tries to do to help support people so that they don't become as vulnerable to the sects, or to bring them back into the Church."

"There is a problem of our own culpability in this situation," Padre Tomas said. "There would not be the success that they've had if there had not been a huge vacuum within the churches. Historically, in our churches, there's been a problem of community, and these sects give a theme of community. We were too theoretical, too intellectual, and these sects give enthusiasm and a place for emotions. And we have fallen to a very low level of morality, and these sects are very fundamentalist and very strict in terms of morality. So that if we were able to find in our own churches more vitality, then the sects would diminish."

It Happened to Them Themselves

Someone asked Padre Tomas to expand on the possible collaboration between the fundamentalists and the Pentagon.

"There are several bulletins," he answered. "There's the Rockefeller document. It very clearly points out the strategy of using Protestantism as a way of controlling Central America. And the Santa Fe document is also a strategy that uses these sects." We would have further discussion of Nelson Rockefeller and the Rockefeller report later, when we met with Padre Andres Giron.

"But you know, even when we read that, it's hard for us to understand. Because we think of their bad intentions, and I think that the people of the United States, with clear minds and good intentions, oppose these strategies.

"So the Pentagon, or the government, or whoever it was, decided that to pacify this area we need to put in sects that will transform these people, who have been influenced by a church that has become communist."

I was shocked by the idea that not only did the powerful of Guatemala think the Catholic Church was a hotbed of communism, but that the U.S. State Department and our foreign-policy makers thought the same thing.

Later I realized I had no way to know what people actually thought. Thoughts are private. But, opportunistic manipulation is something else.

Padre Tomas continued, "Up in the mountains, the military are saying to those [refugees] who are coming back from Mexico, 'Don't come back to pick up your Bible, because that was the cause of your problem.' That's because they're convinced that this will pacify the people.

"The United States has a grand obsession. Any form of democracy that is different from theirs is seen as communism."

The room was quiet. I wondered why cultures had to be destroyed, why religion had to be used as a narcotic and a means of control, and why religious organizations and clergy would allow themselves to be seduced into such a game of power and control.

"Could you explain the changed position of the bishops?" the priest who was traveling with us asked.

"The Catholic Church and also the Protestant churches have had many, many deaths. In the beginning, the hierarchy, when someone was killed, said that was because he got mixed up in politics."

Padre Tomas paused. When he had our full attention, he went on quietly, "But then when someone very close to them got killed, they discovered that was different.

"Another factor in the Catholic Church was the death of the cardinal. The cardinal was very closely related to the government, and he divided the episcopal conference very seriously. And today the leadership doesn't have this, and that makes it much easier.

"A bishop from El Quiche had to leave the country. Another bishop, who is actually the brother of Rios Montt, didn't leave the country, but he did leave his diocese.

"It happened to them themselves, the repression."

Bishops fleeing their country or diocese apparently reminded him of the forty thousand Guatemalan refugees in Mexico, and he began to talk about them. "Their problems are very similar to the problems of those who are displaced within the country, those who are hidden in the mountains, and those who are hidden outside our country. I think all of them are hidden. The situation is not secure enough for them to return.

"I have a friend. He can't go back to work again. Yes, he can come back into Guatemala and nothing would happen to him, but if he went back to where he was from, his life would be in danger."

It Was Crazy

Someone asked, "Do you feel your life is in danger by talking to groups like this, and what kinds of things are priests doing or saying to get themselves assassinated?"

The question sent strange vibrations through the room. Perhaps it was too personal. Perhaps the answer was too obvious.

"There are things you shouldn't talk about, that are dangerous — the land, and the culture. And I think we put ourselves in grave danger if we begin to talk seriously about land ownership."

Padre Tomas shrugged just slightly. "But just talking to groups like this, I think maybe not. I don't think they're going to kill a priest today just because he speaks.

"But they could do it."

I thought back to his answer when, in August 1989, I heard that he had gone into exile.

"And if you were to organize around these untouchable topics—land ownership," he shrugged slowly and gestured in a way that suggested one's life would be in severe danger.

"They killed priests in the past. Everything that they thought was favoring the guerrillas, you had to get rid of it. Many villages were completely destroyed.

"It was a disaster. It was crazy."

For the first time his tone changed. He whirled his eyes toward the ceiling and gestured as though throwing away something he could not deal with. It was beyond him, incomprehensible. But even in his dismissal was a sad acceptance that some things just cannot be understood. His gesture spoke volumes. He seemed almost relieved to be able to throw it all away with that simple gesture and statement: "It was crazy."

The room remained quiet for some time. I was relieved to hear him say it was insane, because I hadn't been able to understand much of what I had heard and seen since arriving in Central America. Now I felt it might be all right for me not to understand. Maybe it couldn't be understood. Parts of it, at least the more horrible parts, may never be understood.

Poorest of the Poor

After a while, I asked if he would talk about the orphans, and he said slowly, "Probably even a more severe problem than that of the orphans is the problem of the widows. In indigenous culture, a widow is more than abandoned. An orphan always has another part of the family to receive them, but the widow is more isolated. Aunts or uncles will receive a child who is orphaned.

"In the beginning, there were actions by the churches to gather up the orphans. That program has disappeared. Because on the one hand they were given care, but on the other hand they were taken out of their cultural environment.

"The problem of the widows is much more serious. We think there are forty-five thousand widows here. These are indigenous women who have lost husbands because of the war and violence.

"Many of them have had to prostitute themselves. Because it is not understood what a woman is to do without a husband. They don't have the freedom to be independent, as the women in other cultures have.

"My personal feeling about that, I think they're the poorest of the poor, because they come almost asking as a beggar.

"They don't know how to work in an international forum. They're just beginning to organize. They have to struggle against their own hunger, and they are perhaps the people who will be listened to the least. Just the other day, the president said the Christian Democratic Party had more widows than there were widows of the violence. The only difference, which they forgot to mention, is that those widows of the Christian Democratic Party have a salary.

"I think it's the group that has suffered the most. And I think that group should be the priority for the churches.

"Five years ago even, the Church couldn't have helped them, because of the old strategy. If I was the wife of a dead person, I was the wife of a guerrilla. Then I would be guilty also. You couldn't give charity to a subversive, which a widow was.

"Right now, people who help widows are not as strongly condemned. But they still do have problems.

"The priest from El Quiche, he talked to us in the last few days. He had to leave two months ago, and that's because he celebrated a special Mass for the widows, and this is interpreted as returning to the situation of eight years ago."

In the early 1980s, any sign whatsoever that anyone might be supporting or sympathetic to the insurrection was lethal for the suspected person. Often no sign was needed at all. An accusation, an inference, a remote hint would be enough.

"The hope, of course, is that space opens little by little, and that we would campaign for the idea that not all widows are guerrillas, that many of the refugees are not guerrillas. Many victims of the violence are not causing the violence."

A Sin to Pay It

"Can you point to any company here where you perceive a conscience operating, or any company that we could have leverage with when we go home?" someone asked.

"No," Padre Tomas said without hesitation, and we were stunned into laughter by his certainty. Our reaction embarrassed him a little.

After the laughter subsided, which it did quickly, he said, "No, because by definition those who come here to do business do so to make money because of the system, and the system is that they take their earnings here and they send them to the United States.

"The international market has been condemned by Latin America. Not only is the external debt not payable, but it's a sin to pay it, because it will absolutely ruin our countries.

"This doesn't mean that our own industrialists or farmers treat their workers any better. Personally, as bosses, those who come here to do business may be much more honorable.

"I'm talking on a structural level, not a personal level. For example, if the law says you have to pay four-fifty a day, a good employer from the United States will pay maybe five or six dollars. But that isn't a solution, because with $6 you still can't eat."

Padre Tomas's words left us with something to consider — the human consequences of business decisions. Simple return-on-investment criteria were not enough. The traditional business formula had too little compassion.

Perhaps no one ever really expected the Third World debt to be repaid. International financiers had to have a place to put petrodollars. They found that place in the Third World. Those dollars were used to build roads and utilities so that export industries could send greater quantities of food and minerals back to the developed nations at low prices. And those dollars were used to build resident armies to protect that infrastructure.

Now some people on Wall Street want the loans repaid, without honestly assessing how they can be repaid, and at what cost to the human beings in the debtor nations. Other people wonder if the loans haven't already been repaid with capital flight, with decades of low-cost commodities exported for our consumption, with destruction of the ecology, and with the sweat and sacrifice of millions of peasants.

Family Planning

A young man asked about the spiritual faith resources that would lead someone to take chances, given Guatemala's history of violence.

"Your faith," Padre Tomas said quickly and softly. Then he was silent for a long time. His silence reinforced his simple, profound message. "Maybe that's the most important thing that I'm talking about."

Someone asked, "I wonder if you would comment at all on family planning, birth control, or abortion."

"When you look at something like that, you have to look at it within the whole picture," Padre Tomas said. "Remember, we're talking about this situation here in Guatemala. The problem of family planning is a problem really of second order.

"The thing that we most strongly try to defend is that [it should be] the family itself, or the indigenous culture in which they live, who decides freely how many children they will have.

"Within the indigenous culture, we know there are massive sterilizations without asking. It happens. The woman gives birth, they sterilize her, and then afterwards they tell her.

"There are those who interpret our problems here as overpopulation. That our policy here should be to have fewer births and that would solve the problem.

"That would be a policy from outside coming into our indigenous culture, which they don't know anything about. That would begin to destroy that whole culture. It's not a theme that's being preached much within the Church."

I learned later that some people feel Guatemala is a rich country with poor people. For them the issue isn't the size of the population; it's the distribution of the country's wealth.

GAM

Someone asked, "Does the Catholic Church support the work of GAM?"

"GAM has been so discredited," Padre Tomas said. "They let them speak. They let them go out into the streets. They let them go out into the country. But they will never let them present their proofs. They will never be before the court. It's another example of our Western democracy, where you're able to speak out on something, but nothing happens from it.

"Within the new counterinsurgency policy, talking about the disappearances is taboo.

"Land, and what happened in the past, the violence, anything that happened in the past is taboo. And so GAM is going directly against that strategy of not talking about the past. Because they want a condemnation of those who did those acts, and that sounds like what's happened in Argentina. And they're not going to have a repetition of Argentina here.

"Our president repeats many times, 'Look to the future. Let's leave the past.' "

A woman asked about the advertisement against GAM in the morning newspaper.

"This is another tactic we have learned from you, as North Americans. There are a lot of phantom groups, like Fighters for Peace, that sometimes come from the United States or are support-ed by the United States. These names sound very nice," he said, meaning the titles that these phantom organizations adopted.

"It was shameful what they wrote. They were 'fighting for peace,' but they have morally condemned the women. They sign themselves as Fighters for Peace, but they are promoting war.

"I think legally that document is libel. A few days ago another one, very similar, came out against the refugees in Mexico, say-ing that they were guerrillas, that they shouldn't participate in the national dialogue, and it was signed by another phantom organization."

Elephant and Fly

"If this will help you, I think that trips such as you've come on are very fruitful. I realize that North Americans living in North America find it very difficult to understand what is happening here.

"I don't know if you saw the movie *Disappeared*?"

He was corrected by a few people who guessed that he was talking about the movie titled *Missing*. It was clear from the slip where his thoughts were.

"It was made by you, here in Guatemala. And no one believes it. Here it is the same."

It was an important point. Credibility. Even if the facts are stated—the thousands of victims, the million displaced people, the tens of thousands of refugees and widows, the two hundred thousand or more orphans—people still may not believe the facts. The deadly *D*'s, distancing and denial.

Bendfelt used a lower number for the orphans, but he included only the earthquake victims.

"You can't understand it," Padre Tomas said about the last decade of violence in Guatemala. "It's hard to believe that the human race has come to such degradation and commits such horrible acts.

"In our own churches, we have the same problem. There are people who just can't believe. They won't believe it until it happens to them. I understand that people of North America can't understand a situation like Central America.

"My hope is in our faith, because the faith of each person, and within our churches, can't help but give us feelings. And these feelings will give us solidarity, and there will be more lines of communication, of credibility, of brotherhood, sisterhood, that would be above nationalism.

"I think that our faith needs to go above and beyond our nationalism, because nationalism doesn't even appear in our doctrine. That's a political thing of just the last few centuries. The injustice of one country to another, I think, can only be condemned from a universal faith of brotherhood and sisterhood."

Padre Tomas seemed to know that we needed time to think about his last few words. He stared at an empty chair near the wall. When he spoke again, he softened the mood. "A few days ago a friend of mine said to me—The president of the United States, if he's going to govern us, how come he doesn't ask for our vote?

"I think you've got homework. I'm personally convinced that as long as the Pentagon has not changed its mind, these small countries of Central America will not be free.

"Nicaragua will be competely strangled. Not by arms, but by the economy. There's an economic government outside of Nicaragua, stronger than Nicaragua. And the same thing will happen to the rest of the Central American countries as long as North America doesn't give her permission.

"You can be the little fly that stings that elephant in the conscience of your country. We depend on each other mutually, whether we want to or not.

"So I say thank you very much for coming."

Guerrilla War

As we drove to our next meeting we were silent. For some reason, I remembered a moment from the time when I was in boot camp in the Marine Corps, at Parris Island.

One of the obstacle courses that recruits had to master was called the confidence course, and one of the most challenging obstacles was a ladder that went straight up into the air. I don't remember how high it was, but it was high—maybe fifty or sixty feet.

The higher you climbed, the farther apart the rungs got. By the time you got to the top rungs, you had to shin up the side poles, because you couldn't reach from one rung to the next. As I climbed, I thought that maybe this was what it was like trying to get to heaven.

Most recruits tried to get up and down the ladder as quickly as possible, because it was frightening. Some even tried to sneak back down without going to the top rung. I'm not particularly brave about heights, but when I reached the top rung, a feeling of calm came over me. I sat on the top rung and gazed out over the swampy landscape of Parris Island and thought it was beautiful. For a moment, I had climbed above the struggle.

I wondered now, riding in the van, how many Guatemalans would be able to climb above their struggle.

I don't know exactly what I expected to find by going to Guatemala. My years in the corporate world hadn't prepared me for the realities of the Third World, and especially for the realities of a country like this. What I found in Guatemala was war.

When we think of war, we think of soldiers and bullets, bombs and casualties. Inflict the most casualties, you win. Destroy the enemy's will to fight, you win. Build the most and the biggest weapons, you win.

Some people think the good guys always win. They can build the biggest guns because they're the best. Many people thought that way until the Vietnam war, and maybe one reason we were so upset about Vietnam was that those simple, almost romantic notions of war were challenged and found to be grossly wrong.

If we define a war as a conflict in which more than one thousand people are killed in a year's time, over twenty wars raged in the world as 1988 came to an end. At the end of 1987, twenty-two wars were being fought. Those twenty-two wars had resulted in some 2.2 million dead, each one of whom was made in the image of God. Over eighty percent of those victims were civilians, and most of them died from lack of food. There is no time to feed people when armies are fighting.

Economic and Cultural War

There is war in Guatemala: death and suffering; widows and orphans who could tell our leaders and their own about war if the leaders would ask, which they never do.

But the war I found in Guatemala was not just a war of bullets and bombs, not just an army fighting guerrillas. Other dimensions of the war are less obvious, less bloody, but just as cruel.

There is an economic war. The bullets in this war are titles to property, and laws, and ideologies. If the rules are too lax in the economic war, the winners win big. If the rules are too strict, almost no one wins except the rule makers. Regardless of the rules, those who lack privilege or opportunity are the losers. They are not just left to their own resources, to pull themselves up by their own bootstraps, as our culture romantically suggests. They are defeated by those who control the resources.

There's no time in this economic war to discuss things. Time is to be used for harvesting, controlling, and getting more. If one predator doesn't act, another will, and the issue is getting there first. There's no time for poor people, dying children, and widows. Call them guerrillas and move on. Call them subversives and move on. Kill them if necessary, but move on. Don't take the time to talk to them, even during a national dialogue. There is more to be gathered in, and too little time.

The van rolled on to our next meeting. Even we didn't have time to pause and think about Padre Tomas's remarks. We had to hurry on.

There is also the war of bullets and bombs. There is the war of economics. And there is the war of cultures. The winners of bullet war and economic war believe they have the superior culture. They believe themselves smarter, more courageous, more disciplined.

Whenever peasants are killed in Guatemala, the dead are called Marxists, or subversives. But I learned that these so-called subversives are often catechists, reformers, or hungry people whose children are dying of starvation.

Many Guatemalans just want to be left alone to carry on their traditional customs and beliefs. They want to wear the clothes their ancestors wore. They want to raise their children, worship their gods, and speak their languages in peace.

Some indigenous cultures tie the hands of their infants together at birth as a sign that the child is never to use those hands to take from others.

Some believe that the earth is a part of life, and is to be respected.

Some believe that family extends widely; that it includes the neighborhood, the village, the community.

Others think those beliefs are dangerous. It's harder to take from a community than from an individual. They think there is only one God, and that is their God; that there is only one set of rules, and that is their set of rules; that there is only one way of doing things, and that is their way of doing things.

They are frightened, so they kill. They are reminded that they might not be right, so they kill. There may be too little to share, so some must die, and some must have their culture destroyed. Or perhaps they can win without killing, so they destroy the other culture instead.

In Guatemala, there is a war against the indigenous culture. It is a war to drive people from their land and teach them new languages, new customs, and new values.

Religious War

There is also a war of religions in Guatemala. This was, to me, the most shocking discovery of my trip — the combat waged by one church against another, and by one faction within a church against another. Progressive Catholics are struggling with conservative Catholics. Fundamentalists are struggling with traditional denominations.

In the United States, we believe in the separation of church and state, but that separation is one of the great myths of our culture. They cannot be separated, unless there is no place for morality in politics. We expand upon that myth to suggest the separation of morality and business as well. But that separation cannot be made either. Business is not amoral. Neither is governing.

So we pretend the separation exists. We tell enough people about the separation for a long enough period of time and some of them come to believe in it passionately. They come to think that the separation is one reason we are superior.

Then we ship our beliefs to others. We tell them how to do things. Guatemalans are being told to use religion, instead of bullets, to keep things under control. So much for the myth of separation.

We help them set up the resources and programs needed to make that happen. If anyone resists, they are called subversives.

So Catholics are subversives in Guatemala. Catholics are communists in Guatemala. So are traditional Protestants.

There are wars going on in Guatemala — wars of bullets, economics, culture, and religion. Lethal wars, wars that we fuel with our greed, our ideas, our resources, and our labels.

These wars have been going on for decades, and they are inten-
sifying. They pit the mightily armed against those armed with
sticks. They pit the wealthy against those who starve. These wars
must be stopped or surely they will spread. Walls cannot be built
high enough or strong enough in our shrinking world to contain
them.

Labels, partial truths, prejudices, and greed must give way to
a willingness to discover and to a worship of what's possible, to an
openness of mind and a thirst for civilization's growth.

The van kept moving through the crowded, smog-filled
streets. What would Padre Tomas be doing tomorrow, or next
year? How would the women of GAM keep fighting? I thought
about the movie *Missing*. I wondered if anyone would believe me.

———————

War, like peace, is the result of something else.
War is the result of selfishness,
of self-centeredness,
of false illusions that violence solves problems.

Peace is the result of love,
sharing wealth,
forgiveness.

There is a negative peace, based on fear.
There is a positive peace, based on trust.
A negative peace is the peace of Herod.
A positive peace is the peace of Jesus.

Colman McCarthy
Center for Teaching Peace

———————

No other place in the world
is as colorful and hospitable as Guatemala.

Color is everywhere,
from lush, green foliage, tranquil blue lakes,
to the multicolored costumes of the inhabitants.

Add to this setting a background of eight million smiles,
as seen in the faces of Guatemala's people,
and you now have the picture—
a paradise of color and friendship.

Travel Brochure
Guatemala Tourist Commission

4

The Palace

High Spirit and Strong Respect

The National Palace stands majestically before a large square in Zone One of Guatemala City, a gray-green stone building famous for its neocolonial architecture, its enclosed patios, and its paintings, murals, and decor. It's also famous for being the scene of numerous coups.

On the palace's left is Guatemala's eighteenth-century cathedral, known for its statues and paintings and for a bronze black Christ.

Directly across the plaza from the palace are retail shops in a colonnade that reminded me at first of the Rue Rivoli in Paris, although that impression evaporated quickly as memories of the Tuileries, the Louvre, the elegant hotels, and the Parisians themselves came into my mind.

As I left the shops and walked across the plaza to the government center, what struck me were the people standing in front of the two famous buildings. In front of the palace were dozens of heavily armed, crisp, polished soldiers. In front of the cathedral were beggars.

We were guided into the palace and through the security checkpoints one at a time. Our bags were searched and our passports checked carefully and kept, to be returned when we left.

The hall and the staircase we ascended were dark, as was the large receiving hall we entered to wait for our meeting. When the lights were turned on in the hall, we saw that it was beautifully appointed. We had only a short time, however, before we were ushered across the hall to a large room for our meeting.

We were met by a secretary in President Vinicio Cerezo's Public Relations Office, Arnoldo Baetz Caal. He seemed to be a warm and pleasant man who genuinely liked people from the United States.

Baetz began cheerfully. He was happy to have us in Guatemala. He had worked with Peace Corps volunteers in years gone by, he said, and "I remember, very tenderly, my relation with these young people helping our country."

Baetz was convincing. I didn't doubt that he was recalling pleasant times with good people.

"I worked for four years with two or three groups of volunteers from the United States, and for me it was a very interesting experience because they came with a very high spirit, to know our culture and to live with our communities. They were learning about how the people live or work in the rural areas and in the small towns."

He remembered the Peace Corps people working in impoverished conditions, he said, with little water and poor housing, but always they retained their "strong spirit." He spoke of his gratitude to President Kennedy. "In his memory, we say always that the United States was, and is, and will be, very near with the countries of Latin America." The United States, he said, "will be" a close and good friend.

Baetz thanked us for coming to Guatemala. Too few North Americans knew about his country, he said, and about the progress it had made. Or about its beauty and history.

"We speak twenty-three languages. Not dialects; really languages, perfect languages," he said.

Television cameras started filming us, and Baetz told us it was nothing, just a little film for the evening news. As the cameras rolled, we introduced ourselves as an ecumenical group. Baetz smiled and made some general comments about how important churches were to Guatemala.

He said he was Catholic, but noted that other churches were "working very, very good" in Guatemala. "We have very, very strong respect for the Evangelic or Protestant churches here."

Esquipulas

A group member asked him to describe what she thought was growing cooperation among the nations of Central America.

Baetz responded that there was more cooperation, but that "never before did we have problems of the magnitude we face now. No one ever imagined the intensity that the problems here would reach."

With this, he captured my interest. I hoped he would explain why the problems were so much worse than ever before, but when he tried, I felt he was giving just a fraction of the truth.

He said things started to change significantly in 1960, when the Central American Common Market began operating, and foreign investment increased.

The Common Market was supposed to create jobs and promote commerce among the participating countries, but within two decades it fell apart. Baetz claimed the demise was due to Nicaragua's "change of political style. Prior to that, all of the countries here were what we would call liberal democracies." Liberal in this context meant that foreign powers were free to invest and own.

Baetz's Spanish was a steady, fluid monotone, and our translator's voice was equally mellow, which sometimes clouded the drama in Baetz's comments.

Nicaragua began to owe large sums of money, Baetz said, and Common Market trade was impaired by its defaults. He neatly avoided any discussion of ideologies or political interference in each other's countries, leaving Nicaragua as the villain simply because it didn't pay its bills.

Without pausing, he moved into a related subject, saying that as soon as President Cerezo took power in 1986, he initiated activity to create a Central American parliament. The parliament was to be a place where common problems could be discussed and resolved.

Baetz took great pride in the Esquipulas treaty discussions, and especially the fact that the Esquipulas II documents had been signed "in this very palace" on August 7, 1987.

He recited some of the provisions of the agreement: there was to be a dialogue with opposition sectors in each country; a national reconciliation commission was to be created in each country; an amnesty was to be declared for members of all opposition groups, political or guerrilla. The idea of a Central American parliament was approved by all the participants but Costa Rica.

And there he stopped. He said no more about the troubles Central America faced, or about the relationships among the countries in the region, or about the peace process begun with the Esquipulas II treaty.

He did not discuss which Central America countries had been best at complying with the peace accords. He wanted us to believe that Guatemala was a leader in such compliance. I learned later that that was not the case.

Reconciliation

"The principal objective for the Guatemalan government of Vinicio Cerezo is to continue working to strengthen peace," Baetz said. "And we will not rest from that until peace has been obtained."

By now, Baetz had lost some of his credibility in my eyes. He seemed sincere, but what he said lacked depth, and other members of the group seemed to feel the same way. We were polite and attentive, but I saw few notes being taken, whereas in other meetings we took copious notes.

Baetz said Cerezo had traveled recently to the other Central American countries to remind his peers of their commitment to peace. "And we are confident that although the process will not be easy, and will have many difficult steps, we have taken the first important steps to carrying out this process."

A young man asked Baetz, "How has this administration decided which opposition groups to dialogue with and which ones not to dialogue with?"

The question gave Baetz an opportunity he seemed to have been looking for. He said it was an important question. "It is not the government that is going to invite different groups to come and sit down at the table," he said. "The government is one of the groups that will sit down at the table."

He was asking us to believe that the government was powerless in implementing a major provision of the Esquipulas agreement, which only a minute before he was talking about with pride.

He said it was the National Reconciliation Commission that decided who would be invited to the dialogue, and the commission was composed of opposition political parties, the Catholic Church, an "honorable citizen" at large, and the country's vice president. He emphasized that the person in charge of the commission was the Catholic Church's delegate. "In a few words, then, the commission is absolutely independent."

Padre Tomas and the leaders of GAM, of course, disagreed.

Human Rights

A woman asked him to talk about human rights. She'd heard that improvements had been made, she said. Baetz seemed glad to respond affirmatively. The most important thing, he said, was that the Cerezo administration had the "political will to respect the life and physical integrity of people.

"The constitution states that the purpose of the government is to look for the common well-being. So all the government's actions should be aimed at promoting the well-being of the human person and strengthening the destiny, and the future, of that person."

He said the new constitution provided for a human rights ombudsman, who "looks out for and protects all persons and their human rights." He said there was no such thing as political repression or persecution in Guatemala under Cerezo, and that the United Nations and other international organizations had recognized the great improvement, "although there is still much to be improved upon."

Baetz's pace didn't change, nor did his tone. The words were neither convincing nor antagonizing. Maria Emilia Garcia's sad gaze came vividly into my memory.

"The majority of human rights violations now have to do with common crime, or common delinquency, which takes place in any society," he said.

"It may seem a paradox, but precisely because of the protection of human rights, a man can no longer be detained without a written order of the judge, unless he has committed a crime at the moment he is apprehended. And the police are often very frustrated by this, because they can't operate as freely as before."

Pornography

"One of the themes that I would like to speak about with you, because of the nature of your group, is the freedom of religion. No one is persecuted for their religious beliefs. Rather just the opposite. We believe that religious conviction is an important ingredient in the moral health of the country. We believe that the church plays an important moral role.

"You may not realize that Guatemala has a cable television system, and we can see almost any television show that's available in the United States."

He had my attention now. I wondered what this had to do with human rights.

"And many things are beyond the control of the goverment as far as the kind of material that's offered over the television. Many times we wish there were ways for us to prevent some indelicate things coming to us. Such as pornography."

Eyebrows went up throughout the room. I could almost hear them bang against the high ceiling. He had challenged us. He had displayed some of our dirty linen. We were asking about their human rights record, and here he was talking about our pornography.

The roles and relationships shifted instantly. We were no longer the judge and jury. He was no longer the defendant, and he knew it.

"Or the violence that is shown so much in television movies," he said.

When he was sure we understood his message, he changed pace again. "But we believe it is the family that offers the best protection against this distortion. And people like yourselves, who believe in God, can help to strengthen the family to help provide this protection."

He had knocked us down and then he picked us up. He was good. He was in public relations for a reason.

Coup Attempt and Kudos

After we had recovered a little, a woman asked about the coup attempt. Baetz must have answered this question a hundred times before, because he moved into a patter that made me think his tongue was turned on while everything else was turned off.

No shots were fired, he said. It was a lack of discipline. The military took care of it quickly. A few officers gave a bad order and a few soldiers obeyed. By early morning it was over. Much overblown by the media. Cerezo didn't even invoke his emergency powers.

Tourism was important to Guatemala, and it was increasing again. The government wanted no sensationalism in the press. The officers responsible had been pardoned.

"There were no changes in the government as a consequence of this movement."

I asked if the government was satisfied with media coverage of Guatemala. I might have known he'd say nothing negative about the media, and he didn't.

"We believe that the work they carry out is very professionally done," he said. "It's very objective. And they are truly professional journalists." Then he recalled several recent media events, including the visits of foreign government dignitaries.

"One of the most extraordinary series of events that has happened during the nearly three years of this administration was, first, the arrival of nearly sixteen thousand peasants demanding land.

"Then, after that, the demonstrations of union workers demanding an increase in their salary. And a series of demonstrations that have taken place in the plaza here, right in front of the palace. All carried out peacefully.

"The minister of defense is an extremely capable man, who, together with other high-level officers, is convinced of the need for Guatemala to continue with the democratic process.

"We have to remember that the army was the government for many years. It was the army, very intelligently, who initiated the return to constitutional government."

No Conditions

Someone asked if Baetz expected any change in relations with the United States under the Bush administration.

"We have seen the example of elections in the United States," he answered. "It is a very inspiring kind of example–stimulating. Because we are trying to carry out democracy, build democracy. And so we want to have our people see how other people live under democracy.

"In recent years, the United States has begun again to sell weapons to Guatemala, after many years of not doing so. But not lethal weapons. Spare parts for helicopters, automobiles, and jeeps, and that is increasingly important."

He did not elaborate, but he did say, "There are still a few centers of guerrilla activity with which the Guatemalan army needs to deal." Then he modified that by saying, "We think that the guerrillas are no longer a danger."

He added that he hoped for continued U.S. aid. Guatemala needed AID assistance and help with its foreign debt, he said.

"If there are changes, the changes will be positive, such as more people like yourselves coming, who can see the poverty, and can see our needs so that programs based on cooperation may increase and bring positive change.

"The United States has never, at any moment, placed conditions on its economic aid to Guatemala."

The comment seemed to stand by itself—a request, or a demand, or a threat. Something flashed in Baetz's eyes as he said it. It was the only moment when his demeanor wasn't entirely calm and warm.

The meeting was over. He had challenged us at the right moment; the meeting had stayed calm; he had been gracious about all the groups loyal to the government; he had sidestepped the painful issues. And only for a split second did he seem to lose the warmth and sincerity that had marked his bearing throughout the meeting.

We thanked him for his time. A young man added piously, "We're especially pleased that this administration is so concerned for human rights, and for the welfare of the poor, and for the participation of all sectors of society. And finally, I hope that each one

of us can be a good influence in our country, so that we can be good
neighbors to Guatemala."

I was glad when the young man sat down. I had Baetz's challenge about our own dirty linen in mind.

In spite of two and a half years
of civilian government,
Guatemala remains
one of the worst human rights violators
in the hemisphere.

The improvement has reversed itself in the cities.
And in the countryside,
there's a de facto military dictatorship.

Nothing has changed.

Anne Manuel
Americas Watch
November 1988

Many times it is impossible to prove legally
that a certain individual is a communist;
but for cases of this sort
I recommend a practical method of detection
— the "duck test."

The duck test works this way:
suppose you see a bird walking around in a farm yard.
This bird wears no label that says "duck."
But the bird certainly looks like a duck.
Also he goes to the pond
and you notice he swims like a duck.
Then he opens his beak and quacks like a duck.

Well, by this time you have probably
reached the conclusion that the bird is a duck,
whether he's wearing a label or not.

Richard C. Patterson, Jr.
U.S. Ambassador to Guatemala
1953

5

Padre Andres Giron

Pro-Land Peasant Federation

Most of us were glad to leave Guatemala City and get into the countryside. We knew the scenery would be beautiful — the foliage, the majesty of the volcanoes and mountains. It was Thanksgiving morning, 1988.

Not a small thing either was the clean air. For people from Minnesota, the air in Guatemala City was foul and difficult to breathe, full of dust and pollution. Most of us suffered at least mildly from sore throats and burning eyes.

Guatemala City's population has exploded. In 1976, the earthquake resulted in a major increase. But that influx was small compared to the arrival of refugees from the violence. Over one-third of the country's population now lives in the capital city, which is located in a valley, an ideal setting to trap the pollution that spews, for example, from thousands of old buses.

But it was not just the scenery and the fresh air that made us glad to leave the city. We wanted to visit with Padre Andres Giron. Padre Andres was one of the few outspoken advocates for land reform left in the country.

We had been told more than once that several topics were taboo in Guatemala. The first item on that list was always land reform. Talk about it even quietly and privately and you put yourself at risk. Talk about it openly and you sign your death warrant.

Still, from his parish center in a small village in the agricultural lowlands of southern Guatemala, a village called Nueva Concepcion, Padre Giron had nurtured a movement advocating agrarian reform, and in spite of the danger it faced, that movement had become strong. In May 1986, Padre Andres led a five-day march from Nueva Concepcion to the capital. Some ten thousand peasants participated.

By February 1988, the movement had grown from scattered groups across the country into a consolidated organization called the Pro-Land Peasant Federation, with a membership of some 150 thousand.

You Give Us Force

The names of many Guatemalan villages begin with *nuevo* or *nueva*, meaning "new." Most of them have been built, or rebuilt, since the violence of the early 1980s.

It was no surprise, therefore, to see that Nueva Concepcion was a series of neatly laid out, relatively new, small block houses. Nor was it surprising to see that the dirt roads we traveled coughed up clouds of dust, or to see children in tattered clothing, or to see dogs, pigs, and chickens roaming free.

It was no surprise, either, to see well-armed military patrols throughout the village and the surrounding countryside.

Padre Giron joined us on the porch of his modest home. He wore a white cassock and glowed with a warm, friendly smile.

He is Guatemalan, but a little taller and stockier than most. He has a commanding presence, comforting yet powerful. I liked him immediately, and he greeted us all as though we were old friends. Birds sang joyfully in cages on the porch, and I felt at ease.

"Welcome to this country. I hope I do well in my English," Padre Andres said.

He sat in a rocking chair facing us and joked, "I'm losing my English." We laughed gently, introduced the group, and outlined the items that we wanted to hear him discuss—land reform, the pastoral letter, the coup attempt in May, the recent attempt on his life.

"First of all," he said, "I think having people like you in this country, for us, is a great privilege. Because I think you give us a lot of force, just coming to visit us."

He said people were watching him, and watching us. People from both ends of the political spectrum. He said several times that people coming to visit, people showing an interest, were extremely important.

"Your presence gives us a lot of security. This is one of the most important things."

I felt uncomfortable again, and very far from home. That gnawing discomfort I had felt when I first saw the military patrols had never left me, but now and then it became more acute. This was one of those moments.

Very Communist, You Know

Padre Andres said that Guatemala was a "tiny country," but growing very fast. By the year 2000, its population might exceed fifteen million people. People were starving in the country now. The need for some kind of change was obvious.

Guatemala could feed that many people, he said, but the ecology would have to hold up. Exports would have to decrease. Land use would have to change. And the country would need help. The U.S. had sent a billion dollars to Guatemala so far this decade, but I saw few signs that the money was making much difference.

"It's incredible to see the necessity for land reform," Padre Andres said. "Seventy percent of the land belongs to one percent of the people of this country. We do believe that, in this country, there will be no social changes until we have some justice as far as land is concerned."

He said that he and some supporters had started to work aggressively for land reform about three years before. "But it has become a very political issue—extremely dangerous and difficult."

Some reform activity had taken place under Cerezo. Through the government's Agrarian Transformation Institute, eight farms had been sold to peasant organizations since late 1986. The land was purchased by the government, then sold to the peasant groups through low-interest, long-term loans. Padre Andres's movement obtained its land this way.

But getting the land and developing a plantation were only the first steps. After that, the property had to be protected and the crops sold.

The government's land reform program was limited by the financial resources available to acquire land and then finance its purchase by the peasants. The Guatemalan government just didn't have a lot of money for this purpose.

Padre Andres said his group had four plantations now. "And we are presenting a new structure of work. We are trying to see if we can work collectively. And that means very communist, you know.

"It really means, well, this priest is trying to create communism inside this country. So I'm a dangerous person for that."

He smiled as he threw out the label. He seemed to want to defuse the fear of communism by using the word openly. For Padre Andres, labels didn't mean much. What people did was what had meaning.

One Goal

"Our movement has one goal," he said, "to change the economic and political structure of this country."

Peasants had no voice in running the country, and illiteracy was a major problem. "Eighty-five percent of the people are illiterate."

Even if land were given to the peasants, there would still be many problems, he said. Technical and business training was needed, and money to develop the land and markets for its products.

"There's a lot of ignorance here. It's not because they want to be ignorant, but the structure of our society has made them ignorant."

Padre Andres seemed to become self-conscious at that point, perhaps wondering if our group was classifying him with the illiterate Guatemalans. For just an instant, his face revealed some doubt about us. He seemed to wonder what prejudices we brought with us into his patio.

Meanwhile his birds sang, chirped, and laughed at all of us for our heavy thoughts and sagging spirits. Bible passages don't come into my mind often, but the music of Giron's birds caused me to remember one: "Look at the birds of the air: they neither sow nor reap nor gather into barns, and yet your heavenly Father feeds them." I promised myself I would think about this passage more carefully later.

Padre Andres said that they were working their plantations in two ways. The large operation was being run collectively. However, smaller projects and homes were owned and managed by individuals.

In 1987, the crops had been good, but the harvest "was burned by some people from the private initiative." Estimates of the damage place it at more than twelve thousand dollars; the average Guatemalan family lives on less than two hundred dollars a year.

Amnesty

Padre Andres said he was constantly asked to do things for people. He did the best he could, but the things he was asked to do were difficult and dangerous. A few months before, an attempt had been made on his life.

He said the government blamed the guerrillas for the attempt, but he didn't believe the guerrillas were responsible. The government even "put some guerrilla movement guys in front of the TV and newspaper, and they were saying that Padre Andres was protected by the whole guerrilla organization of the whole country." And I was giving them food and uniforms.

"And honest to God, I haven't done anything like that."

Amnesty was supposedly provided to opposition members under the terms of the Esquipulas peace agreement, he said.

"So right now, the rightist people, the people who have the money in the private sector," Padre Andres said, "they are saying that if I'm a guerrilla I must go into amnesty, which is totally wrong for me.

"So I told them,'Why don't you go, because you are the killers.' I really told them, very, very strongly.

"And so they told me they were going to take me to the judge, to the court. And so I said, 'Okay, I go. And it's the first time you're going to do something legal. You're taking me to the court. Usually what you do is you kill people, and that's it.'"

The Coup Attempt

Then he switched gears and began to talk about the attempted overthrow of the Cerezo government. He said that the powerful wanted certain things and were prepared to get them, one way or another. And they did.

"After that coup [attempt], prices got loosed. They raised prices. They started private initiatives. They start doing what they were asking to do before. So they are the ones who are manipulating the whole thing.

"And, even though you might hear that in this country we have a democracy, I'm beginning to doubt very much.

"This is a simple, pure military show concerning democracy in this country. You know, Vinicio [Cerezo] is not managing this country. It's just a front, a little—what do you call? Marionette. He's not leading this country. And, we don't have a democracy at all.

"After that [coup attempt], the eleventh of May, we have a lot of killings.

"And if you talk about human rights, the killings, it is getting worse and worse every day. Three days ago, they killed about three persons not too far away from here. And nobody knows. After the eleventh of May, we lost about four people within our movement. One was shot to death, and another was disappeared, and we don't know yet where he is. And two others were killed."

His voice trailed off. The porch became still. I felt myself changing—I didn't know from what, or to what. Just changing. Softening. Grieving. Then he began again. He said the violence was becoming as bad as it had been at the peak of the violence in the early 1980s, except now it was more sophisticated, more "covered up."

Someone asked him to expand on what he had said about how

they worked the plantations. He repeated that communal work was very important in his mind. He said that if the peasants were given a small piece of land, it wouldn't help them. They also needed money, and surplus crops to get that money. Bare subsistence farming was not enough.

Corn was no longer an economically attractive crop, he said, but it was a deeply rooted part of the indigenous religion. According to that religion, the gods created humanity from corn. The contrast between its economic value and its cultural value was enormous.

Guatemala can import corn from the U.S. and Brazil more cheaply than it can grow it. So the federation's output of corn is of little export value. In 1987, they had seventy thousand pounds of corn to sell. They hoped for twenty quetzales per hundred pounds.

"But the rich guys, the ones who have chickens and all the poultry, they got three hundred thousand tons of corn from your country. So they lowered the prices in this country. And this is the way they play. So we have to sell our corn now for fourteen, fifteen quetzales a hundred pounds.

"And you have to pay for your fertilizer, which is very expensive, extremely expensive. So with the working of the soil, fixing the ground, and putting fertilizer and insecticides and all that, it's impossible to get any good prices from our corn.

"The thing that really gives us food is sugar, coffee, maybe sorghum, a little bit of sorghum, and soybeans, and that's it."

A Fragile Economy

Dependence is a much-used word in Latin America. An entire theory of international relations is built around it. Free-market capitalists suggest that all the Central American countries need to do is what the U.S. and other developed nations have already done: invest, work, raise productivity, reinvest, and repeat the cycle. Eventually this is supposed to raise the standard of living for the entire society. No one explains, however, exactly when or how the investment will be made, or by whom.

As I sat on Giron's porch, I remembered my college classrooms and business boardrooms where the theory had sounded reasonable. Now I wasn't at all sure.

I wondered if another perspective might not be that Guatemala's means of production are too tightly controlled by the elite, and that all the country can build on is its land and its labor. The labor is unskilled, uneducated, and scattered. The region lacks a good infrastructure—roads, harbors, information systems, communications, and educational facilities. It also lacks stability.

Guatemala is not a place for investment, according to this perspective, and without investment the development cycle cannot get started.

The tools of repression—the military, the theory and technology of counterinsurgency—have been developed, however. That's where investment has been made.

The export industry has been developed too. Exports allow the quickest return on investment, and generate profits that can be trapped outside Guatemala more easily than is the case in other industries.

"So we have a very fragile economy," Padre Andres said, "and everything depends on how much we sell to your country and to Europe. I do believe that we are dependent too much, too much, on the countries who are very well industrialized."

He said again that conditions could be improved through agro-industry, but only after something is done with the skewed ownership of the land.

"It will happen when that seventy percent of the land is in better distribution," he said.

The traditional Indian culture had to be taken into account here, Padre Andres said. The Indians were deeply loyal to their heritage of private cornfields on which they grew the corn they needed for their tortillas. The transition from the private cornfield to the large plantation was more than an economic matter, it was also cultural. Giron's strategy was to effect the economic transition without harshly interrupting the cultural heritage. Both changes, economic and cultural, would have to evolve slowly, despite the urgent need to feed the hungry.

But evolution could easily give way to revolution. One assassination in Nicaragua, that of Pedro Joaquin Chamorro in 1978, made all the difference. The same held true in the Philippines.

The Pastoral Letter

Someone asked Padre Andres what he thought of the bishops' pastoral letter on land reform.

"Honest to God," he said, "I think we push for that letter," meaning that his land reform movement was one element that had encouraged the bishops.

He didn't think the letter was radical. "They only say a better distribution of land." He also didn't think the letter would effect much change.

The bishops were trying to be supportive, he said, but he was clearly disappointed that they weren't working more aggressively on the issue. "I don't see a bishop coming into our movement and saying, 'Well what can we do for you; how can we help you as an institution.'"

"It's a nice letter. But that's it." He waved his hands in the air to emphasize the futility of expecting results from it.

Although he didn't say so explicitly, I began to see that the Church was in the midst of a struggle, probably a desperate struggle, between progressives and conservatives, a struggle that some believe could be as explosive as the Reformation was four centuries ago.

"They are trying to take my priesthood away," Padre Andres said. "Right now. They send a letter to the Pope—especially the rightists—saying that I am a communist, I am not performing my duties as a priest, and my priesthood should be taken away."

His bishop had asked him to resign from his two parishes, but he had refused. It was his work.

"I'm trying to do my best. But I believe that, you know, right now we have a very difficult situation with the Church. Our Holy Father is putting people very conservative in the Church—extremely. People who really see that everything is covered up. So we have those problems that we have to confront.

"You may ask me a question—why is a priest getting into that, a political situation?"

He pointed to his shabby church with its dusty wooden benches for pews. It was small, spartan, without murals or gilding.

"Being honest with you, you might see my church is not as nice as you might think." But, he said, buildings have nothing to do with the real Church.

"And I believe that when you preach to people, and when you see that they are not paying attention because they're hungry, it's very difficult to put the gospel within their hearts."

I didn't know much about hunger, not really. I knew even less about hungry people, or a hungry nation, or hungry people by the millions. For me, hunger was an occasional donation, or a television spectacular about starvation in Africa, and after that I went back to day-to-day living, where hunger was not a problem. We never discussed hunger in the boardrooms.

Now I was reminded that empty stomachs have trouble hearing the word of God. I could almost see the empty stomachs of the Guatemalans now. I began to understand that only if you felt through those stomachs could their reality be understood. Reality had to be seen from the inside out, indelicate as that might seem, and that was impossible from a distance.

Martin Luther King, Jr.

Padre Andres talked a little about romance and adventure.

"You know, when I became a priest, I had a very romantic idea. I would be blessing people, and it would be nice. And I would be very well dressed." He smiled at his innocence.

Then his smile went away. "Now I know that it's a huge burden on your shoulders when you really take up your duties as a priest."

He said a Christian had several basic responsibilities. "You are a prophet, bringing the good news to people. And if you are a prophet, you have to fight against everything that goes against the good news.

"You have to offer your life to God, but to people too. And you have to serve people."

He paused for a long time. The birds sang sweetly in their cages. I pondered seriously in mine.

The phrase "good news" was familiar. Since Vatican II, I had heard it used often in Church services. But good news seemed to have a different meaning in Guatemala, especially when I heard it said by a man who was prepared to quite literally sacrifice his life for others. It became a revolutionary phrase, a liberating phrase, a phrase that says each human deserves the same opportunities every other human deserves.

What Padre Andres said next gave me an insight I hadn't expected. He said he hadn't learned about being a Christian in the seminary. "Somebody taught me that. He was American from your country. I had the privilege to work in Memphis, Tennessee, with Martin Luther King, Jr. And he really taught the commitment of a real Christian."

I was struck by the realization that in coming to Guatemala I was rediscovering my own country, and I was reminded that in both Guatemala and the U.S. people were suffering.

Padre Andres said he was a revolutionary when he was younger. He was willing to fight violently for change. "I believe we still have some chances to change this country, not through weapons, but through peaceful means."

I understood by now that violence was never far from people's thoughts in Guatemala. Most hoped to avoid it, but few shrank from it.

"I have done many visits with your Congress people," Padre Andres said. "I have pushed a lot in the United States to see if we can change the policies. Many of the policies, for me, are very wrong. They just think that selling weapons, and putting more force into the army will help the situation.

"I think you can do a great job to change those kinds of policies."

Not long before, we had been told that the U.S. State Department had recently approved the sale of almost fourteen million dollars in new weapons, M-16s, to the government of Guatemala. The transaction was a private deal between Guatemala and Colt Industries, but any such weapons sale requires State Department approval.

I Will Go

"I think we have to change this country," Padre Andres said. "One group wants to change it through violent means. I believe that violence won't get you anywhere."

He said his movement might try to elect people to congress, or to the presidency, to change the laws of the country, which are "really laws for the rich, not for the poor."

Someone asked how he felt about the danger to himself and to others in the movement. He seemed almost nonchalant about it, and took almost no time at all to consider his answer.

"It has become for me a way of living, honest to God. When you receive many threats, you can adjust to it. I believe that nothing will move without the will of God. And when it's my time, I will go." He threw his hand into the air with a gesture of finality, as though he were tossing his soul into another world. "I will go."

I was stunned again. Padre Andres was willing to die for the poor. No one I knew was willing to die for a business deal or quarterly earnings, although I knew a few who were working themselves beyond reason. In fact, I knew a few who had literally worked themselves to death in the business world.

I realized we all die for something. We all die for the answer to our First Commandment question—who is our God? Padre Andres just had a different answer.

"So right now, I have this historical moment," Padre Andres said.

I knew it would take me a long time to digest what Padre Andres was saying. Service, sacrifice, and a sense that our lives were moments of history: these concepts felt good, in tune with values that softened my heart. I felt I was experiencing an historical moment of my own. And I wondered if my friends would understand what I meant if I told them about it. I wondered if I myself would ever understand entirely.

When Giron's historical moment almost came to an end, just two months before, it was "a horrifying moment," he said. "You don't think about yourself. You think about the others who were injured. I never thought about getting hurt. I got real mad. And I went to the guy, and I said 'What have I done to you?' And I put my arms on one of them."

Then he paused and his anger evaporated. We were not going to hear more about what happened in the attempt. What happened after he grabbed the man? Did his anger need to be checked at that moment? At this moment? Why did he end his story just when he put his hands on the man?

When he began again, his voice was peaceful and composed.

"And being honest with you, I do believe that if we are Christians we have to believe in His word. Nothing will move without the will of God.

"So, whenever is the time that I should go, I will go."

The attempt on Giron's life was not without impact, however. People became even more frightened, he said. Some quit the movement. I wondered if that wasn't the real objective of the assassins — not to create a martyr, but to frighten his followers.

"They are scared now with the radio and TV and everybody saying, 'Well, Padre Andres is a communist.' The same in your country. They are afraid of it. I don't know why the United States is so afraid of the communist threat. If people are well fed, well educated, with a little chance of a future, you don't have to worry about that."

Someone commented that communists don't believe in God. Which God? I thought. The money god?

"Yes," Padre Andres said gently. "They think communists will put God into prison."

Rockefeller

I asked Padre Andres to talk about the mix of religious denominations in Guatemala, and about the declining proportion of Catholics.

"That was a contribution of Nelson Rockefeller," he said. "Maybe you remember, your vice president when Gerald Ford was your president. He came to make a tour to Latin America, and one of things he said was that one of the most evil things were forces that we have in the Catholic Church. Because it's the only institution with credibility in Latin America; the only institution. So we have to divide it."

The idea that the U.S. interferes with not only economic and political matters, but with religious ones as well, was difficult for me, as was the idea that officials of our government think of religion as just another tool for control and domination. It wasn't naivete; I just didn't want to believe it.

Since my return from Guatemala, I have studied Rockefeller's involvement. The Rockefeller family has had business interests and investments in Central America for years. Nelson Rockefeller's own business interests there dated back to the 1930s, and he was well versed in the affairs of the region.

President Nixon asked Rockefeller for advice on Latin American affairs, even though he and Nixon had been political rivals. In fact, Rockefeller traveled to Latin America four times in 1969 to review conditions before making recommendations on U.S. policy.

Some of Rockefeller's report seems to me to have made sense. He wrote: "I think they find themselves very much in the position which we did at the period of the Continental Congress in 1776, and . . . what we rose up in arms against the British about, we are now doing to the other Western Hemisphere nations."

Rockefeller went on to predict that "we are moving rapidly into a period of revolution."

Since the beginning of the Alliance for Progress program in 1961, he noted, there had been seventeen coups d'etat in Latin America. This instability was the primary barrier to progress of any kind. Stability could best be achieved through military means, not a restructuring of economic and political distortions, Rockefeller reported.

Out of Rockefeller's recommendations came the Nixon Doctrine of 1969. It declared that the U.S. would no longer serve as the world's policeman. The U.S. would instead work "realistically" with those regimes that had the capacity to maintain order. Stability was to be our first priority in foreign relations, regardless of what kind of conditions were stabilized.

Thus in 1972, when the average Guatemalan peasant earned just over eighty dollars per year, the U.S. sent almost seven million dollars in weapons to that country.

The State Department also began an active program of encouraging the missionary work of fundamentalist churches in Central America. The theory was that if the peasants focused on the hereafter, they would be more likely to accept the conditions of the here and now. The Catholic Church had filled that role for centuries, but as elements of the Catholic Church became progressive and active in sociopolitical and secular programs, a void had been created.

Jesus Is Very Cheap

"In this parish last year, we had forty-nine churches," Padre Andres said. "We have now fifty-two. And one Catholic church. In this area!"

The situation in his parish was consistent with what we had observed elsewhere. Everywhere we saw small churches—in village huts, in clearings along the roadsides, in dilapidated houses in the slums. From them all rang joyous music.

"They are selling religion very, very, very cheap. Jesus is very cheap for them. You know, you raise your hands, you're safe." He was referring to the alignment between the fundamentalist churches and the military. One way for a peasant to avoid violence was for them to join a fundamentalist church.

We would be told elsewhere that the members of these churches were often the ears of the military. From them intelligence was gathered on any possible insurgency, on revolutionary activity, on efforts to improve living conditions.

"Besides that," Padre Andres said, "you know, they are very fundamentalist. They believe in what is written, and that's it. There is no tradition. They are teaching an evangelical Jesus, who is in heaven. And what they tell the people is that you don't have to worry about the evils of society. Don't worry about it. You are poor, and keep poor.

"Now Marx is very right when he said that religion was the opium of the people. It could be. It can really make people zombies. People without will, without anything. You know, they just clap their hands. They go wild. You know, they have great music. Real sentimental. And religion is not sentimental."

I have fundamentalist friends, and I thought about them as we traveled through Guatemala. They're good, caring people. It was difficult for me to understand how different denominations could come to oppose each other so bitterly, or how they could go to such extremes. At what point does goodness and caring become perverted? I realized that the question had wider application.

Loaves and Fishes

"I believe in one miracle that really changed my mind, and my life," he said. That was the miracle of the loaves and fishes. I was beginning to think I was on familiar ground when he shocked me again.

"To me that's a big lie," Padre Andres said, referring to the idea that Jesus created an enormous feast from a few scraps.

"It's more truthful when you think that Jesus came up and talked to people, and he knew that people were hiding bread. And he had the power to convince them that you must share your bread with others. And that's when the miracle happened."

I had heard a homily on Luke 18:25 just a few months before coming to Guatemala, and I remembered it now: "For it is easier for a camel to go through the eye of a needle than for a rich man to enter the kingdom of God." It's a difficult passage for a pastor to explain to a flock of wealthy U.S. Christians.

The eye of the needle always intimidated me a bit, and I had tried to ignore it. In Guatemala, the eye of the needle became an invitation to read more of the New Testament. I wondered what Rockefeller thought about the eye of the needle.

The idea that it was a miracle to persuade people to share—that was new to me, and sad. But I was beginning to believe in miracles again.

"The greatest miracle," Padre Andres said, is "if you can change the suffering of people. If you can change that, then this world will be better.

"And if we can take all the Catholic and Christian teaching, and we really go into the real deep witness of the word of God, it really makes you free. I do believe in that. It really makes you free.

"That's why my preaching is not just blessing. I scream, and I yell, and I do whatever I can do in order to tell the people, 'Look, you are going to be a Christian. Christianity is not for the people who want to live their life comfortably. It's a pain in the neck.'

"Honest to God, I do believe in that. To be a Christian is not just to say the Mass, but to invite the world to be in the real Mass, in which everybody can share what they have, especially their life.

"Theology of Liberation is a way of life here. We live it.

"Maybe you have passed your exodus in your United States. We are beginning our exodus to a new land, to a new promised land. And this is our hope.

"That's why maybe a priest is a little crazy. But I think, if you find Jesus — I found Jesus in a different way. Not with music, but with a real justice for the people. There I found Jesus."

A Great Adventure

Padre Andres told us he had received his master's degree in sociology in Memphis, and felt very proud of his diploma.

"One day they invite me to a Mass. And I thought these people are stupid, you know. I was coming from the States. Look at their faces, so simple. I said, well, what the heck. Here I am, I know more than they. Look at them, the stupid people, singing.

"But there was a lady who had a beautiful kid, with a huge head like this," his hands shaped a disproportionately large head. "And his smile." Padre Andres paused. "And that smile changed my life, being honest with you. I thought, you know, I knew everything.

"I knew nothing in those days. I didn't even know Jesus."

I thought I understood. Children's smiles had always warmed my heart. I was thinking about how profoundly important children are when Padre Andres interrupted my thoughts with an insight that made my entire trip to Central America worthwhile.

"To be a Christian is a great risk, but a great adventure. To me it's the best adventure I ever had in my whole life."

I felt then that I knew why I had come to Guatemala, and I wanted to stop right there. I wanted to go home and explain to my wife why I went to Guatemala, and what adventure really meant.

But even when life-changing discoveries are made, other people go on, and so did Padre Giron's homily.

"And that's why I like this mess. I will continue to bother the rich, and to bother the rightists, and to bother your government. I will continue to do that," Padre Andres said. "Even if I have to give my life.

"I'm just telling you what I feel about it, and what my convictions are. If we want to change this world, we must share what we have. Especially your life, which is the most important jewel that God has given you."

A Chance to Be

"The Church has quite a lot of power," Padre Andres said. "Lots of it. But it's not using that power for the people. It's using that power to maintain itself. You go to the Vatican, same thing."

He had gone into a three-year exile for his safety a few years earlier, and he was invited to study at the Vatican.

"And I quit. Being honest with you, I just could not stay in Rome. Jesus came to serve, not to make shows."

A member of the group echoed, "To make shows."

Padre Andres said, "Yes. And I don't like that."

Eventually someone asked the inevitable question — what Padre Andres hoped we might do when we returned to the United States.

"Push your government to change their tactics. I think people like you can really make a big difference, if you can make your people conscious.

"When I went to the States the first time, they asked me where Guatemala was located — young kids. And they asked me, 'Father, did you ever ride in a car?'

"And I say 'No, this is my first time.'

"They say, 'How do you do it in Guatemala?' "

He said he told the children, "You know, we go totally without clothes and hop from one tree to another."

Our group laughed a little self-consciously.

"But a year ago, I went to Los Angeles, and I saw people from the States walking in marches, and talking about Nicaragua, talking about Guatemala. A new spirit is coming up in the States, and this is our great hope.

"So I think you're doing great. Just coming to this place, for us, makes us stronger. You really make me strong. Even in the States, my actions, and the actions of people are ringing.

"And we are in the same boat.

"If you can tell people that here there are people who love too, the same as you. There are people who need to eat, who need to be educated, who need to be well, with good health. People who are people. I think that would be the answer.

"I think many people think, 'Well, you are a *spic*. You are a little down, you know.'

"I remember, when I was in the States, they always talk to me like 'you are a spic.' That I had the speech of a spic, when I came up. I didn't know nothing about anything, and I went right into the university. Six months later, I was teaching. And I was a good student. And I tried to do, to be, my best.

"There was a lady who taught me logic. She was a nun. She said 'Your negatives and my negatives are different.' And that was a big problem for me. One time I said, 'Would you, sister, explain that to me again?'

"And she told me, 'You better go fight with the guerrillas. You are stupid.'

"But I didn't care."

For the first time, I didn't believe him.

It was time to stop. Padre Andres left us with a last thought.

"I can tell you one thing. We are capable. You know, the poor people are intelligent. They are not stupid. If you give them the chance, well, they can do it.

"I think, in this world, people are looking for a chance—a chance to be."

A Chance to Live

After our visit, I learned that in December 1988, Padre Andres Giron announced that he would be a presidential candidate in the 1990 election. Some people have said he has a death wish. Padre

Andres responded, "If my life has a chance of changing this country, then I'm going to do it. Then my death will be worthwhile."

Death is no stranger to Padre Andres. He receives death threats constantly. He escaped an attempt on his life in September 1988, when thirty men in military uniforms fired at his car while he drove down a dusty road near his parish in Tiquisate. His bodyguard, Leon Velasquez, was killed in that attack. Giron's adopted son, Fernando Castellanos, was wounded.

His father, who was a town mayor and provincial senator, was killed in 1981. An aunt and three other members of his family were also killed in the violence of the early 1980s.

On May 27, 1989, CBS broadcast a segment on Padre Andres, called "Father Revolutionary," on its *West 57th Street* program. Steve Kroft introduced the segment by saying, "Our next story tonight is about the kind of man we usually don't hear about until after he's dead, killed for challenging those who have the power and the guns. He's a priest and he's very much alive.

"For most of the last decade, he's lived under constant threat in a country that is one of the most brutal in the world. Guatemala, a loyal U.S. ally in the fight against communism, also has the worst human rights record in the Western hemisphere.

"But it may be a measure of how things are changing there that we've managed to find him before a bullet has."

In December 1988, Padre Andres said, "They think I'm a communist. I'm not. But I'm not a capitalist. I think both systems are evil. I think we have to create a new social system where people have a chance to live, not only survive.

"Carrying a gun is not my style, but when you are not able to do anything legally, when you find yourself against a hard wall, you think about it."

We recognize that in the final analysis
the most difficult thing is
personal conversion.

Conversion means a "turning around,"
a radical change.

As long as one's only goal is profit,
to grow rich,
ambition for money or power,
it is impossible to understand these truths
which we have desired to bring to mind,
and to see with Christian eyes
the reality which must be transformed.

"The Cry for Land"
February 1988

The human being, every human being, is
— God's beloved creature,
— made to His image and likeness,
— endowed with intelligence and will
and therefore called to be free and live in community.

Moreover, every human being is called by Christ to grow,
so as to become a sharer in the divine nature,
and thus reach full realization in God.

This is the source of the immense dignity
of the human person.

1976 Pastoral Letter
Bishops of Guatemala

6

San Lucas Toliman

Thanksgiving

The temperature dropped as we drove to higher altitudes on our way to the mission of San Lucas Toliman. We had left the smog of Guatemala City behind us; now we were escaping from the dust, humidity, and heat of the Pacific plains.

Everywhere we looked was beauty—mountain peaks, green foliage, plantations ripe with coffee. The roads were crowded with Indians, men walking with packs of firewood on their backs, women with jars on their heads. Occasionally we saw a mule loaded with cargo. Often the men carried machetes and hand tools to use in the fields. Most of the men and all the women wore indigenous weaving, and the colors of their dress added to the abundant beauty of the countryside.

Now and then the scenery was marred by a military patrol— eight, ten, sometimes two dozen soldiers in green, U.S.-type uniforms. They held their weapons ready, and I found them intimidating.

The road had two lanes, and wound its way through the coffee plantations up to Lake Atitlan. There it climbed and went around the east side of the lake to Solola and we turned off on a side road, one lane and dusty, to San Lucas.

We drove just a little faster than the Indians walking beside us. Only a few of them looked up. We had passed no vehicles since leaving the lowlands, and even in the lowlands we saw few vehicles.

It was late in the afternoon when we bounced along the main street of San Lucas Toliman. We drove straight through to the church and rectory. Just beyond was the lake itself.

Father John Goggin greeted us, and we visited briefly before he led us to the mission's guest house, next to its tiny experimental farm.

The guest house accommodated perhaps twenty people. It had been used by the military as a torture center during the violence, and it felt like a barracks. We were told not to drink the water. The shower trickled cold water when it worked at all.

After stowing our gear, we went back to the mission for Thanksgiving dinner.

The rooms that were home to the mission's three priests adjoined the old church. They were small, comfortable rooms, and we ate in the largest of them, which served as both dining room and den.

It was a happy time for all of us. We had been traveling for almost two weeks, and San Lucas Toliman seemed like an oasis in a terribly troubled land. We were glad to be there.

The meal was as festive as any Thanksgiving dinner I'd had at home: turkey, dressing, salads, vegetables, potatoes, bread, milk, cheese. We were introduced to the cooks, four women in local dress who smiled as they acknowledged our applause.

Still, I felt more than a twinge at the unfairness of our feasting while others nearby, just outside the door perhaps, had too little to eat. I'm no Bible scholar, but later I ran across a passage in Amos about despising feasts. It didn't seem to fit this meal entirely, but it reminded me strongly of rich, business-related dinners I had attended.

I thought about guilt, but I didn't feel guilty. There was often a subtle but fierce struggle for dignity at business dinners too. I felt everyone was searching for dignity, and that was a larger issue than guilt. Still, it was impossible to dismiss the unfair distribution of the fruits of God's earth, and there was reason to feel guilty when guns and torture were used to maintain that injustice.

We finished our meal and visited for a time. Then the group began to break up.

I wandered through the village for a while, looking at the stars above the glistening waters of Lake Atitlan, and worrying about the eerie thumping sounds that echoed through the darkness, the sounds of mortar shells bursting on the other side of the lake. Soon I found myself going back toward the church, joining a stream of San Lucas people, men and women, headed the same way. The thumping sounds gave way to the toll of the mission's bell.

The church held few things of elegance, and that made it supremely elegant and comfortable. There were a few pews in the front half of the church, a few pictures, fewer statues. The old-fashioned altar, which was from the colonial period, was almost hidden in a chapel-like enclosure.

Between the altar and the rest of the church, the wall turned inward to provide a frame for the choir screens that used to separate the lower-class faithful from the wealthy faithful so the two would not have to mingle in the house of God.

The men sat on the left side of the center aisle, the women on the right. A catechist directed the prayers and singing.

I sat on a bench toward the back of the church, turned on my tape recorder, and was soon surrounded by children, as intrigued by the blinking red light of my machine as I was by what the machine was recording. The singing had a fervor that was as honest as anything I had ever heard.

Father John Goggin

Father John had agreed to meet with me later in the evening, so after the church service we began our visit. Father John had been at the mission for twenty years. He's a gentle man and was a gracious host. He spoke lovingly of going out into the hillsides, to areas that can be reached only on foot, to say Mass and teach and help the people in whatever way he could.

One of the mission's priests, Father Greg Schaffer, who founded the mission in 1964, was resting in Minnesota, and in his absence, playing host to a group from the States was awkward work for Father John. He seemed uncomfortable much of the time.

I asked him about life on the surrounding plantations. The system dated back to colonial times, he said. Workers had always been needed, and they were brought in from the highlands. Often the

owners built shelters, and communities developed that were completely dependent upon the landowners. The plantation workers
looked to the owners for food, education, health care, and religious
support. "They would have to go and get a priest to come and celebrate the one Mass a year, and to build a chapel, and things like
that," Father John said.

Today, he said, the trend was away from such communities.
"The plantation owners have not been interested in maintaining
that structure much more than they have to. They would prefer to
work with migrant labor," which left the people even worse off.

I learned later that one major reason for preferring migrant
workers was that the migrants were harder to organize into unions
or recruit into guerrilla bands.

Some of the plantation communities were many years old.
Many generations were buried on the land. "In our parish, the plantation owners still maintain and allow the people to live on the
plantations for the time being, and they work there."

But the people wanted their own land, he said, and it was impossible for them to find it. Land cost a thousand dollars an acre
when it was available for sale. A plantation worker earned a little
over three quetzales a day, about a dollar and a half.

Studies indicated that a family needed a minimum of sixteen
quetzales just to sustain life. They were earning one-fourth of what
they needed. My mind turned briefly to Bendfelt's bus drivers.

The families were all large—six or more people. "The people
would have tortillas, which is corn baked over an open fire," he
said. Perhaps they would find some greens along a river, and from
these they would make soup. And they would always try to have
beans. "That would be the main things they would have." They
might have salt, coffee, maybe an egg, "and possibly, once a week
or once every two weeks, some kind of meat in soup. It would be
an ounce of meat and some fat per person. Meat is extremely expensive."

How many families, I wondered, had ever even seen a meal
such as we had just enjoyed.

When the mission first came to San Lucas, Father John said,
there was great hunger, so they began their work around that problem. The missionaries helped the people grow vegetables to supple-
ment their diet.

Then the mission concentrated on helping the people own their own land. Support from the diocese of New Ulm, in southern Minnesota, provided most of the funds. Two small colonies of a few hundred homes have been started in recent years.

"In fact we're going to bless some of the houses there on Saturday. We planned that there'd be something like two acres for each person to farm." But there just wasn't enough room for people to live, and the land for farming had to give way to land for living.

"The people just don't have any place to live," he said. Even the most generous plantation owners were no longer building shelters for the people. Young families were building lean-tos attached to the huts of their parents.

"Of course, then the problems of families living so close together are really difficult."

Education

If the people have no land, the plantation is supposed to provide education for them, Father John said.

"But once they live on their own land, then they become part of the national education system. They can go to a public school run by the government."

I asked if the plantation owners were good about providing education. "We've had really good cooperation in our area with the plantation owners about promoting literacy," he said.

At the mission school, the Sisters of Notre Dame worked with Guatemalan personnel. But there were too many students. Interest in education was very high. Besides operating the school in San Lucas Toliman, the mission sent twenty teachers into remote areas. Sometimes the plantation owners paid the teachers, and some plantations even provided incentives for the children to remain in school and wouldn't allow them to work if it interfered with education.

Guatemala's level of literacy, Father John said, was one of the lowest in the hemisphere. He thought half the people couldn't read or write Spanish. Perhaps seventy-five percent of the men were literate; of the women, ten percent. More of the young were literate.

Not many years ago, he said, the plantation owners used to say, "The people have the trees and the sun and don't need anything else. They can work the ground. That's their lot in life."

"I think the people felt that way about themselves," Father John said. "And that's where the gospel comes in.

"That's so important, that people realize their own dignity, realize their own dignity as sons of God, realize their own dignity as loved by God. That God thinks highly of them. That He considers them His own people. And Christ is a brother.

"Once they can really appreciate all that, the positive things from the gospel, then they have a much better self-image. And they start demanding some of the opportunity to realize their potential."

Bishops Called Communists

The San Lucas mission grew out of a discussion between two bishops attending Vatican II. "Bishop Melotto buttonholed all kinds of different bishops, including Bishop Schladweiler, to staff these parishes," Father John said. Bishop Schladweiler was the first bishop of the New Ulm diocese, and in 1958, I had been his first crosier bearer.

The mission had not survived without terrible sacrifice. Father John described some of the struggle the mission had survived, and how the people felt about that struggle.

"The poor person, the person who has no strength or anything, is caught between people who feel that they can solve things by power, by being strong and coming down hard on one side, on the right. Or by being on the left and saying, 'By raising up with might and arms, you're going to throw off oppressors.' So between the two situations, the extreme right and the extreme left, you have the people who are being crushed, for no reason at all."

The people weren't political, he said. They had no confidence in politics.

"They would like to be able to live in peace and run their small plot of land," he said. "They're not asking for a lot of money, or anything like that."

Of the four women who had cooked our Thanksgiving feast, he said, three had lost their husbands.

We were silent for what seemed a long time.

Then we talked about the children in the mission's orphanage. They were from homes where no one could care for them, Father John said. The parents were dead, some of them from starvation. He wouldn't say how many were orphaned by the violence. Starvation was the biggest killer. At least one hundred orphans lived at the mission.

I asked about the bishop's letter on land reform. He said it wouldn't have much impact.

"The bishops have been called communists. Everybody who's a communist is bad. You put a title on people, and that automatically discredits them."

He thought it was a good letter, and an extraordinary action for them to take.

"It takes a lot of guts for them to talk about it."

They've Given Life

We began to talk about the members of the New Ulm diocese.

"The people in New Ulm," Father John said, "they've given life. They've shared their life with people down here. The changes over these twenty years are really notable, and are really, really tremendous changes."

The giving ran in two directions, however, he said. The poor gave to the rich as well.

I thought of the power I felt listening to the music in the mission's church. I had much to learn from the lives and values of the San Lucas peasants.

"These people can only depend on God," Father John said, "and they do depend on Him." For their future, for what's going on, for what they can hope for. And the response from the diocese of New Ulm looks to be the hand of God in their lives. I think it is.

"It's also the hand of God in the lives of people in New Ulm. Somehow we all have to become poor to let God work in us."

The New Ulm diocese contributions, he said, had "made it possible for people, so many people, to have new opportunities and new life. People who before never even had the opportunity that one or two children might live, now can see children with university educations."

One young man was about to become a lawyer, he said. Three or four were about to become doctors. The school was now staffed almost entirely with San Lucas people. The doctor in the mission clinic was from San Lucas, as was the entire mission staff. He was proud of that.

Cattle Ranches

Speaking of the people of San Lucas, he said, "Competent they are. Initiative they have. Creativity they have. They learn quickly. They have an insatiable, continuous desire to learn."

The people had one day off from their work on the plantations. That day, Sunday, was generally used to gather firewood, go to the market, or work their plot of land, if they had one.

Yet when a catechist was teaching, they came from miles away to study and learn, and would do so for weeks, until the course of education was completed.

Their feeling about the land was strongly spiritual, he said. One of the nearby plantations offered them corn at a reduced price, about a third of what it usually cost, but the people preferred to grow their own corn, even though it required a great deal of work, and might even cost more to produce than it would to buy.

"But the people have to be producers," Father John said. "The people, from their history, have to grow corn."

Often growing their own corn meant walking great distances, and working marginal land. But, Father John said, "That makes them feel like a human being. Corn is sacred. Corn is something that at least retains their dignity. That they're producing something with their own hands for their family."

San Lucas people seldom ate meat, he said, and they seldom got enough protein. Yet meat was a major export crop. The cattle were grass fed, so a lot of land was used for grazing.

The highlands were all dedicated to coffee. So the people had to go to the lowlands to grow their corn. They rented land on the cattle ranches and cleared it to pay their rent, or they plowed up pasture land that had hardened from grazing. There they planted their corn, planting grass between the rows just before they harvested the corn. They got a small corn crop, and the owner got new grassland for the beef.

Safer to Be a Fundamentalist

By now the others in the group had finished their wandering and joined us in the den. We were tired and ready to turn in, but someone asked about the fundamentalist churches we had seen in both Honduras and Guatemala.

Father John said it all began with the Rockefeller report. Things had changed considerably since the days when the Catholic Church was a partner of the establishment.

"The Church would be the normal rallying point for the poor" if everything were going the way it should, he said. "But if you can divide the poor among themselves, and have them fighting and worrying—about passages of the Bible, whether your people should have processions and saints, whether honoring the saints is bad and people that have processions are bad, and all these customs that people have had over the years—then you don't have people being united."

He said some people joined the evangelical churches because of their stress on not drinking. Some joined to avoid contributing to the community and the Church.

"During the heavy times, when there was so much violence, we didn't use the word 'catechist' in our talks. A catechist was considered a guerrilla, a Catholic guerrilla. In some communities, people would become titular Protestants during those years, because they didn't want to endanger their lives. It was safer to be a fundamentalist."

Then we adjourned. It had been a full day. I made a mental note to ask Father John about the picture of a young man, nicely framed and placed on a small bookcase in the den.

Father Stanley Rother

The next day, I learned from Father John that the picture on the bookcase was of Father Stanley Rother. In 1981, few news stories reached the U.S. from Guatemala in spite of the violence. What few stories there were, however, were about a priest, Father Stanley Rother, who had been murdered just a few miles from San Lucas Toliman.

Father Rother had been warned to leave Guatemala as the violence grew, and in 1980 he did. By that time, thirty people from his village, Santiago Atitlan, had been either murdered or disappeared. He left grudgingly, because he had worked among these people for thirteen years.

But then he returned. He told his family, "If I have to die, I will die there. I want to be there with my people."

In July 1981, he was shot by three men wearing ski masks. He was the ninth priest, and the first from the U.S., to die in Guatemala in 1981.

Friends who knew him maintained that he had always been careful to avoid politics. He was conservative. Said one, "He was the real low-key type, just doing his job. His real delight was upgrading the agricultural and health level of the people, training and teaching them."

The Reagan administration had been in office only a few months when Father Rother died, and its ambassador-at-large, General Vernon Walters, had visited Guatemala only one month before to try to induce the government to improve its human rights record so the U.S. could restore aid.

President Lucas Garcia gave specific orders for the killing to stop during the Walters visit. But immediately after Walters left the country, the death rate soared to record levels.

The Rother murder slowed the Reagan administration's efforts to supply lethal aid to Guatemala, although jeeps, trucks, and parts began to find their way into the country. To accelerate the flow of aid, the Guatemalan government announced that three suspects had been arrested in the Rother killing.

The government alleged that Father Rother had died trying to prevent a robbery, although friends argued that he wouldn't have risked his life for the few worldly possessions at the mission. The government said eyewitnesses had identified the men. One eyewitness was Sister Ana Maria Gonzales, a Mexican nun who had been sleeping in another building at the time of the killing. A nurse from the U.S., Bertha Sanchez, another witness, had also been asleep. Both women fled Guatemala immediately.

A dead priest's picture on the shelf of a bookcase, malnourished children fighting to stay alive in the mission's clinic, beautiful people singing their hearts out in a small seventeenth-century church, volcanoes rising majestically over the water of Lake Atitlan, soldiers patrolling the streets and mortar shells bursting on the other side of the lake, a festive meal, a gentle, loving priest—these are some of my memories of Thanksgiving in San Lucas Toliman.

Troops were stationed permanently in San Lucas Toliman after we left. In August 1989, three guerrillas were killed in a shoot-out a few hundred yards from the mission church.

In November 1989, Father Greg Schaffer, who was in Minnesota for several months, asked me if I knew any groups who might want to hear about Guatemala. I telephoned over a dozen churches and talked to the pastor or to the social-justice program people. I called on several in person. In each case, I either knew the pastor personally or was referred to the church by someone with a personal connection. I called several personal friends—one was the president of one of our state universities; another was a member of the board of regents of a Catholic college.

My efforts were fruitless. None of the churches or schools wanted to hear about Guatemala from Father Greg. Some thought he was looking for a handout; some thought they knew all about it already; and some were just too busy.

———————

The thief comes only
to steal and kill and destroy;
I came that they may have life,
and have it abundantly.

I am the good shepherd.

The good shepherd
lays down his life for the sheep.

John 10:10-11

———————

These people will not accept
this kind of existence for the next generation.
We would not; they will not.

There will be changes.

So a revolution is coming—
a revolution which will be peaceful
if we are wise enough;
compassionate if we care enough;
successful if we are fortunate enough—
but a revolution which is coming
whether we will it or not.

We can affect its character;
we cannot alter its inevitability.

Senator Robert F. Kennedy
May 1966

7

Milpa

The Health Clinic

Early on Saturday afternoon, November 26, we were to meet a man in the parking lot of a health clinic in a town I shall call San Pedro. He was several hours late. We had been told that nothing could be said about the man or about "what went on there," so we didn't ask. We were concerned, but we trusted the judgment of our guides.

Most of us thought of what was planned as a social outing, a chance to spend the night with a peasant family in Guatemala—to eat their food, see how they lived, experience real poverty if only for a few hours. Our conversation touched on our supply of blankets, whether it would be cold sleeping, what food our hosts might serve, how we would communicate. Those who spoke no Spanish hoped the family would have children, so that the universal language of peek-a-boo and tickling could ease the passage of time.

Across the dirt road from the clinic was a compound. Perhaps it was for patients, or once had been. It was another thing we didn't ask about. Around the compound was a stone fence; above and attached to the fence was a wire-mesh fence. The mesh was covered with sheets of black plastic to prevent anyone from looking in.

But the standard Guatemalan diet of beans and tortillas doesn't promote growth. The men tend to be a few inches taller than five feet. The women are barely five feet. And the plastic barricade had been made with Guatemalans in mind.

What I could see was that the compound had at least four block buildings, sleeping quarters which, with bunk beds, could each accommodate two dozen men. Three dozen if they crowded. At the south end were smaller units, able to hold four or five people, quarters for nurses, perhaps, or supervisors, or leaders of some sort. I wondered if this was a military compound.

At one point while we waited, I heard men's voices singing, a large chorus, but not singing out fully. Church music accompanied by the muffled clapping of hands. Then the singing stopped suddenly.

Family Problems

When the man who was to meet us came, he explained that he was late because of "family problems." He was calm and spoke freely, gently. But his "family problems" were not the kind I associated with calm, or with gentleness.

Twenty peasants had been disappeared two days earlier. Eight of the men were from one family, and several of these were his brothers-in-law, husbands of his sisters.

Late yesterday, one of his brothers-in-law had been found, shot to death. Early on this morning, another brother-in-law had been found, also shot to death.

In the midst of this tragedy, he took time to greet us, saying he welcomed us with love and affection, telling us not to worry, that our hosts were looking forward to our visit, and that we would be received by gentle and kind people. He said he was sorry that he could not be with us that night and hoped we understood.

We had bought a few melons that morning, and these were to be our only gifts. No payments were to be made. No blankets were to be left behind. Such a gift would be too extraordinary, and news of it would circulate throughout the area. It was to be enough that we were there, he said—that we were spending even just one evening with them.

We asked if there was any danger to our hosts or to us. The man said no, and our leaders said that if there were danger they would not proceed, but that it was the families who were at risk, and they would not accept the risk if it were too dangerous.

The man who had come to meet us said he was frightened, that he was a coward. Mary told him she thought he was very brave. We weren't sure what they were talking about.

To Milpa

A guide appeared on foot and visited privately with the first man for a time. Then we climbed into our vans. I rode with Mary and another group member. The man we had met in the parking lot was one of Mary's closest Guatemalan friends, and she began to tell us about him. He had become a leader of the health promoters following the devastating earthquake of 1976. The promoters had tried to provide help to the victims, and as part of that effort, a nationwide organization of volunteer first-aid workers emerged.

With international aid, the promoters built clinics and created a network of health support services, a network that often intermingled with public service projects: agricultural diversification, crop improvement, sanitation, and immunization programs. Sometimes they were affiliated with progressive church groups. Often they worked independently.

Mary's friend worked full time as a health promotion leader in the late seventies. When the violence began, he was suspected of being a subversive, as were most leaders of efforts to improve the lives of the peasants. He went into hiding. A few years ago, he decided it was safe enough for him to live openly.

In the last year, however, he had quit his work with the clinic and the health promotion programs and had gone back into hiding. He had become "much burned," which meant he was identified as a subversive, a risk to political stability, a man whose name was on "the list."

He came out of hiding now and then to help a program or a movement, or to arrange a visit for U.S. travelers with peasant families, or to bury a family member who had been found after a disappearance.

It was "just a matter of when they'll get around to him," Mary said. "He won't survive the next round." Then she cried.

Milpa, an alias I've given the village, was less than twenty kilometers from San Pedro, but the drive took well over an hour. The roads were dusty, rutted, and rocky, winding up mountains and down.

We crossed several bridges on our way. All had been destroyed during the violence. They had been rebuilt and showed the signs of recent construction work. I doubted they had been repaired to improve transportation for the peasants, almost none of whom owned vehicles. The military seemed a more likely beneficiary.

Mary told us that the twenty peasants who disappeared two days before were not the only disappeared in the area. An entire truckload of men returning from working in the lowlands was disappeared a month ago—forty men, all still missing. Not even the truck had been discovered.

Her crying became sobbing. When she could speak again, she said, "It's going to start all over again. They're going to die by the thousands. They're going to slaughter the people."

We stared out the windows and waited for her tears to stop. We watched Indians walking along the dusty road in their colorful dress, the women with baskets and jars of water on their heads, the ever-playful children with their beautiful smiles and wondering eyes. We saw their huts, made of mud, cornstalks, corrugated tin, and stones. We didn't speak.

The Violence

The Milpa area had suffered more than most of the country. Not far from where we would sleep that night were widows and orphans by the thousands.

In Guatemala, over a hundred thousand people had been killed in the violence; another forty thousand had been disappeared. Most were simple peasants. A high proportion were women and children. Now, it was said, the military was using helicopters to drop bombs on the peasants who lived in the area.

"It's starting all over again," Mary whispered to herself.

The guerrillas, Mary estimated, had killed perhaps ten thousand people at the very most and she thought that number was probably much too high, but among their victims were select targets: large landowners, plantation owners, and managers, leaders of the polarized structure.

But the dead are impossible to forget. The powerful of the country had also suffered. Theirs too were painful and angry memories.

At the peak of the violence, the insurgents numbered no more than fifteen thousand, probably closer to ten thousand. Some five thousand of them, at the most, were killed. The rest of the dead, over eighty-five thousand people, were simply caught in between, the alleged and the actual supporters of the guerrilla movement, indistinguishable now. They were mostly the poor, the hungry, victims of a scientific counterinsurgency plan learned from the U.S. experience in Vietnam. The government and the military acknowledge that over four hundred villages were burned to the ground to deprive the guerrillas of their civilian support. Milpa was among them.

A Young Man Speaks

Guatemala, a country promoting tourism, is also a country organized under the strict rules of counterinsurgency. Each community has block groups, with leaders who report to a community military commander, who reports to an area commander, who reports to a department commander.

Within each group, at each level, are infiltrators, who listen for signals of disloyalty and report independently to their superiors, who in turn have their own superiors. Throughout the country there are *orejas*, or ears, as they are called. These ears listen for everything, and report everything.

The orejas are paid. Not much, a few quetzales now and then. When I was in Guatemala, a quetzal was worth less than forty U.S. cents, but in a country where a peasant earns less than two dollars for a ten-hour day of cutting sugar cane, that's a substantial amount of money.

It was clear that few foreigners had visited Milpa in some time. The peasants along the road and the people in the village stared holes into our vehicles. The burnt ruins of the violence were still visible throughout the village.

We slowed to a cautious stop on the dirt main road and tried to turn left toward the shack that our guide pointed out to us as our first destination, but the side street was torn up and full of ruts and rocks. There was room to park only one vehicle.

We left the other vehicle in the main street, where it attracted attention, as did our group as we locked our gear into the vehicles and hurried to the shack where we were to meet. Once there, we discovered that our new host, the health promoter in charge of the projects this office managed, wasn't there.

Instead our guide from San Pedro turned us over to a young man, who sat on a chair in an office too small to garage a standard U.S. car. The guide disappeared as quickly as he had appeared earlier.

The young man was friendly and open. He wanted to know about our weather, and what ice and snow were like, and if our crops were good, and what we grew, and whether it was hard work.

He talked about the crops they grew, and how hard it was to grow them. He talked about religion, and God, and how important faith was to them. He talked about working in the lowlands, and how everyone hated to do that. He said they often got malaria, but they had no choice.

He said he was the man of his household. His father had been killed in the violence. So was an older brother. He and his mother had survived. They would be one of our host families that evening. He apologized for his "heavy eyes that want to go to sleep." We learned later that he and the local health promoter, who would join us soon, had worked through the past night. He hadn't slept in almost forty hours.

Corn and beans were the crops he knew best. These were the most important crops to his people. Now his country imported these staples because the prevailing economic wisdom was that the land was better used for export crops—sugar, coffee, and cattle. The land on which they could grow corn and beans was land that could not be used for export crops. It was land with little topsoil— land on the sides of mountains, sometimes so steep the peasants had to anchor themselves with ropes to keep from falling out of their fields.

The land needed fertilizer. After the violence of the early 1980s, the price of fertilizer was not too high, and the government promised to supply it. But the government's fertilizer often did not arrive on time.

We Work and We Die

"It used to be that if a peasant had land, he was rich," the young man said. "He could grow his corn and beans and feed his family.

"Now even if he has land, the cost of fertilizer is too much. The government and other agencies will lend us money to buy the fertilizer, but then the peasant is controlled in another way.

"The government talks about helping the peasant. It talks about giving the peasant land to grow his corn. But what good is the land if all the crops must be sold to pay the loan that was needed to buy the fertilizer?"

The fertilizer, the young man said, costs thirty to forty quetzales per hundred-pound bag, and one bag covers very little ground.

"If the crop is good, it will feed the family for perhaps ten months," the young man said. "Then we have to find other ways to eat."

Meanwhile, if the family bought clothes once or twice during the year, or if they bought sugar for their coffee, which was bitter because the best coffee was exported, or if they needed medicine, or rope, or a pot, or wire for a chicken coop, if they were fortunate enough to own a chicken or two, the money for these things had to be earned by working in the coffee fields of the nearby plantations, or by going to the lowlands to work in the sugar fields.

If the peasant's crop was not good, malnutrition followed, bringing with it flu, diarrhea, dysentery, and fevers. Then children died faster than the average national death rate of almost sixty percent before age five.

A friend of the young man's came in for a minute, but he was not comfortable talking with us. The young man apologized again for being so sleepy, and urged his friend to talk to us.

"We're really screwed," the friend said. (Our translator may have modified his language a bit.) "The fertilizer is too expensive, so it's no good even if you have land. So you work or you die. You go to the lowlands and you give up part of your life. Work in the lowlands is work that mistreats you, but we have nothing else.

"We work or we die," he said.

"We work *and* we die."

His face had not changed expression. He stared at the floor, with a combination of dignity and despair.

"Hope is the last thing that dies. Hope is all we live by," the first young man said.

"Maybe we can get by, perhaps. For the last two years, they have made promises, but it's just words. They promise fertilizer, but it doesn't come. We buy fertilizer, but the prices are too high. They give something here, but they take away everything on the other side.

"Still, Guatemala is the land of the eternal spring. So we keep our hope."

Massacring Our Own

It was dark by the time the health promoter arrived and exchanged places with the young man. Although senior by just a few years, his posture was that of an older, more serious man.

He, too, had worked through the previous night, and he had just arrived from visiting a project in the mountains. He had walked ten kilometers back to the office.

He wanted to know what kind of group we were, and why we were in Milpa, and what we would do when we returned home, and what we had learned about Guatemala, and whether we believed the government and the press.

We were unprepared to answer questions, and we floundered, but he was patient. I sensed that his expectations, through painful training, were not high. He seemed grateful for any empathy, or any support. Yet he made it clear that these small things were desperately needed.

"The recent U.S. election is fatal for us," he said. "The U.S. wants to defend its patio. The U.S. fights to have its philosophy and its ideals here. It wants to put our people into its framework, its imperialism. These were the policies of Reagan and they will continue, and it will be fatal for us.

"That's just the way it is. That's reality." He shrugged his shoulders slightly.

"Look what's happening. We are massacring our own. We have massacred our own. And we are hiding in U.S. power. You understand it better than we do. You see the world more. We know of these things when we hear of them from others, and when we talk at the market, or as we go about to different places in our work.

"We want to be left alone so we can develop ourselves.

"We have two struggles. We want to open up the lives of people so they can work and live justly. And we have those who want to run everything, and they do it with money and force.

"When towns are working, they call it subversive. Then there are disappearances and kidnappings. And they have weapons that they get from your country and from Israel.

"Heads are cut off. So there is war. Some confront in a nonviolent way. Some fight. But always we live in fear."

We Trust in God

Soon his wife arrived with their two children. She had been with him in the fields but walked back more slowly because of the children. Their little girl was about three. Their son was not yet walking. The little girl had pigtails and a bright smile. She sat on her father's knee as he continued.

"Some hide in the mountains. Some try to live within the law. But always there is pressure from the outside, and from the inside."

We asked about the government programs and the AID programs that were supposed to be much improved since President Cerezo came to power in 1986.

"The government wants all programs to be funneled through it, and if that happens we will never see any of the money," he said.

We asked where his organization received its funds, and he said they came from UNICEF and from humanitarian groups in Holland and Canada.

We asked about his hopes for the future.

"We trust in God," he said.

"When we look at the Bible, and when we look at history, we see that people move ahead only after long struggle. We have just begun here. We will not have what we should have. But we have begun. We do everything possible—while we are alive.

"You can pressure and boycott and influence policies more than we can," he said. "If we do it, it's like killing yourself. So when you visit, it helps us. They might leave us alone.

"There are black parts and there are white parts, and the white part is asking, in decency. Others, from other countries, can pull back the blanket, and we hope you can do something for the people in Milpa. We never want weapons in our hands. We respect life."

Even as he said they wanted to avoid violence, I felt an unspoken threat in his words, a threat that weapons might have to be used. There might be no other answer.

Religion Is Destroying People

His organization, he said, was "the only association in this area with goals to improve production and help the children. This is reality."

The organization had been started fourteen years before, by a group of catechists. After the earthquake in 1976, he and his friends wanted to learn first aid. They studied, organized, and received legal authorization as an organization in 1978.

"At our largest moment, we had thirty coordinators running our programs. But then the violence came and seven of these were killed. The rest of us hid.

"We reorganized in 1983 and 1984. By 1986, we had firm bases in twenty-six communities, and we have many projects in agriculture and health promotion. These projects are the fruits of our martyrs.

"We saw bodies. We saw blood. We were afraid." He stared at a corner of the room, near the floor. "Nature, which is wise, was reborn in us. We are still afraid. But today our courage is greater."

Word came that three of our prospective hosts could not proceed with the visit. They had not received permission from their local military commissioner.

We asked if we shouldn't just leave, but our leaders waved the question off. We continued with the discussion, and asked why he felt their courage was greater now.

"We are used to the threat," he said.

We asked if the women felt the same way, and he said, "Yes, if their husbands explain. We are a part of our history. We cannot stand. We must move ahead."

We asked his opinion of Padre Andres Giron, and he said, "He's a peasant leader. He wants to help the landless. But he has gotten into a conflictive area. Many would like his support. But he is called a puppet, so that his work will lose virtue.

"Months go by, and he's still alive.

"We are not for him or against him. He knows his mission. There is a whole network that distorts and provides misinformation, so we cannot say if we are for or against."

We asked about the Protestant churches.

"In our association, most were Catholics, some were Protestants," he said. "But some non–Catholic fanatics believe social work is subversive.

"Most of those who died in the violence were catechists. Being Protestant protected people from the violence. That's the way it is. We are just little fish in a sea of ideas and policies."

A few of us talked about Protestants in the U.S. We said there were many kinds of Protestants and asked if he meant all Protestants in Guatemala were part of the psychological war. Our host used the word Protestant to identify fundamentalist sects.

"Protestants divide the people," he said. "Catholics unite them. So we have a political problem. And we have a religious problem. Our catechists continue to be threatened. They do it over loudspeakers. They use the catechists' names.

"We don't serve a framed God. We serve a God that is here

among the people. That's how we serve. It doesn't make any difference, rich or poor, but right now politics is destroying people," he
said.

"Religion is destroying people."

Only Killing Demons

The day was getting long for many members of our group.
People began to stand, stretch, glance about. This was no longer a
social outing with a poor family.

There would be no time to play with the children. There might
not be time for dinner. Far worse possibilities lurked at the back of
at least my mind.

Someone asked about the pastoral letter on land reform.

"The bishops' letter says a lot of words," our host said. "But
they are just words. Now the bishops are called communists, and
if there would be more Padre Girons, they would be called the
same. And what would happen is that the priests would be massacred, as in the past.

"Some priests make a commitment to help the people. But
others back off. Some speak with the authorities to help us. Some
do not.

"The Protestants think that development and community work
is subversion. There is a Protestant pastor who talks on the radio,
and he says that everyone who does not accept the gospel, as they
define it, is a communist, especially those who fight for their Catholic faith — they all have demons in them."

Again he was identifying Protestants as fundamentalists because that was his experience.

"After the coup brought Rios Montt to power, Rios Montt said
that he was killing bad spirits inside people — that he was not killing
the people themselves, only killing the demons."

It was under Rios Montt's presidency, in 1982, that the worst
of the violence occurred. Rios Montt implemented Project Ash,
which killed thousands of people between July 9 and July 11, 1982.

"So people became Protestants," the health promoter said.
"That way they could survive the violence. And that has stayed in

their minds. The Protestants are still growing here. In some villages there are three or four opposing Protestant churches. They divide the people.

"Now the Protestants are making war on the people. They say, 'Why work here on earth?' They put obstacles in the way of community work. But we have to move forward. As we are now, we'll continue to work. It will not be given to us. Even if they kill us."

Do Something for Us

By now, we had been listening for several hours. It seemed much longer. The health promoter kept his right hand on the edge of the door, glancing outside every now and then as he talked.

From the time we arrived, there had been music playing on a small portable radio, just loud enough to make it difficult, but not impossible, to hear. I began to understand that the music was to drown out our conversation in case an eavesdropper was outside, and that our host was watching for movement outside the door. All of this was done so easily, so calmly, that it was almost unnoticeable.

I wanted us to move on—to our host families for the night; or back to Guatemala City, smog and all; or back to our comfortable homes and our families.

Someone asked about the families who were not able to have us join them that evening. Why did they not get permission, and why had this man and his young associate received permission?

"The women couldn't come because they didn't have permission," the promoter said. "In every community, there is a military commissioner. Sometimes he is a civilian. People who want to leave or enter or have visitors must have permission or there will be sanctions. This is especially so if the visitors are foreigners.

"Perhaps the women decided out of fear."

What kind of sanctions? Why were they afraid? What had changed in the last month, or in the last few days, that they now chose not to get permission? Why hadn't our leaders known about this change, or about the women not getting permission? How much danger was there?

Instead of asking these questions, we asked about the permission that he had received, only to find out that he had not asked for permission. We were there without the authorization of the military commissioner.

Some group members became quite concerned now. The man explained that this was the only village in the area where permission was not required.

"They won't notice if we go to the homes at night," he said.

I understood now why he had kept the meeting going until it was very dark.

We asked about taking pictures. He said none should be taken. He said he was worried about our vehicles, too. We should use only one vehicle to drop people off at the houses. The other could stay on the side street by the office.

We asked why his village was exempt from civil patrol work. He said they just stopped going. Somehow no sanctions were imposed for this — no disappearances, no murders. But the village was suspect now. They were all watched.

If anyone asked about us, the promoter said he would say that some of us were with his health promotion association and were here to give advice on some of the projects. The others were just tourists who had tagged along.

It sounded lame and made me wonder if our presence here was worth the risk they were taking.

Something outside — some noise or motion — concerned the health promoter, so we sat a while longer. He began to speak even more softly, under the music.

"Our fear has been converted into courage," he said. "But do something for us. There are many eyes."

Twelve Pounds of Corn

The discussion stopped. People shifted in their chairs, or stood. If they had been standing, they sat. I wondered if this man would survive, if he and his village could be helped, if everything he said were true. I wondered if we would have come at all if we had thought the evening would turn out like this. I wondered if anyone would believe what was happening if I told them, and if I dared tell anyone.

"You saw a lot of land growing sugar," the man said. "Yet people starve because they have no land."

There was no need, at this point, for any of us to be reminded. The pictures had become vivid. We had seen children with clear signs of malnutrition. The balding scalps, the discolored hair, the frightened eyes and distended stomachs were vivid in my mind. There were no doubting Thomases among us anymore.

It was still not time to go to the homes. Our group leaders asked if there were any more questions.

Someone said that on our drive to the village we had seen that on the worst turns the rutted surface of the road had been smoothed. Signs announced that the work was paid by the eight percent of the government's budget that had been allocated directly to benefit local communities. When Bendfelt spoke to us, he had seemed proud of this program.

"It's a bribe," our host said. "It's like giving a goat something so it will behave. They give, and then they put their foot down harder. People get no money back, and it's their money that pays for these things. People pay the great debt.

"Like giving land to the peasants. Then they must borrow to buy fertilizer, and use their crops to pay back the loans. It's just another way to keep the peasant down, to keep their foot on his neck.

"We work odd jobs," the health promoter said. "We can earn maybe three or four quetzales a day, if we are fortunate. Then we can buy clothes. A peasant who is fortunate can get different clothes to wear once a year, sometimes twice.

"Or the peasant must go to the coast to work. Then he will lose his health, because the work is bad, and the conditions are bad."

He had worked on the coast each year for fourteen years from the time he was eight, he said.

"On Sunday they give you twelve pounds of corn, three pounds of beans, and a half pound of salt. That is your food for the week. Only the men go to the coast from here. But from some places the whole family goes, and they must live on what they are given on Sunday. Two pounds of corn will make only ten tortillas. Even the widows go to the coast. Or they die.

"We are very small Davids against a big Goliath."

Who Will You Talk To?

"The government has doctors," he said, "but they want too much money. All they care about is money. And the government health center does not respond when it is needed.

"UNICEF training helps, and soon they will give us medicine, and we will have health promoters in over thirty communities next year. We will outstrip the government health centers. But the government is very upset by our work."

We were told later that it was considered subversive to issue a bottle of aspirin to a peasant unless the issuance was part of an official "hearts and minds" government program.

The promoter was wandering from idea to idea now.

"It would be fatal if the U.S. AID money is channeled through the government, like they want. There is no medicine in the hospitals. There is no money for teachers. There are no doctors who help us. But they buy new helicopters. Each day we see these helicopters in our sky. And now they are buying more sophisticated weapons. Why do they need these new weapons?

"The government keeps getting bigger, and it needs more money for itself. And everything is more expensive. It costs ten quetzales to buy enough sugar for our coffee, and soap for one week.

"If you would help us, it would be like a lightning rod for us.

"I thank you for coming," he said. "We told you things sincerely because we trust you and want you to be our friends."

He made me feel that death was imminent; that they would be crushed soon. I thought too about how our lives affected their lives, how what we had—what we took for granted, what we thought we had a right to have—was linked to what they did not have, could not hope for, would not even dream of having.

"There are many tigers," he said.

"How will you summarize?" he asked us. "Who will you talk to?"

We mumbled something about talking to our friends, and maybe some politicians we knew. But we knew, and he knew, that our responses only showed how helpless we felt, and how little we understood.

What would we have done had we been in his place? He remained calm, and his eyes stayed tired and sad. He kept the atmosphere from becoming tense.

"What suggestions would you have for us?" he asked.

We stared at the floor. I mumbled something about keeping faith, feeling stupid even mentioning the word to him. His faith had been tested.

Eleven in Two Huts

At last, we were divided into three groups, one for each of the families who would be our hosts for the night. We gathered our blankets and most essential gear, storing the rest of our things in the office, which would be locked. I worried about the notes we had taken in the last few days.

We drove quietly out of the village, retraced a small part of our journey into Milpa, and headed further up a mountain until our guide told us to stop. We dropped off one party and waited in the dark until their guide returned from escorting them up the steep slope to the hut that would be their quarters for the night. We dropped another party off in the same way. The final three of us stayed with the health promoter, who would be our host for the evening.

We turned off on a small road and discovered, to my surprise, that we had not been driving, earlier in the day, on the worst of all possible roads. It took us fully twenty minutes to crawl a kilometer or so.

Then we climbed through rocks, cornfields, trees, and bushes. We climbed for another half hour or more until we came to two huts nestled in the midst of yet another cornfield. There we were greeted by the promoter's wife, who had left us earlier and walked home with the two children.

There were eleven people in the family, living in the two huts. The promoter with his wife and children lived in one, which included a room in which his two brothers slept. He told us in an almost casual, but still very sad, way that his other two brothers had been killed in the violence.

In the other hut lived his mother and father, a younger brother, a sister, and the daughter of one of his deceased older brothers. We were welcomed into his parents' hut, introduced to everyone, and visited there a short time, warming ourselves by the small wood cooking fire.

Cornstalk Walls

The health promoter's hut was divided into two sections, each no larger than eight feet by twelve feet. Corrugated tin sheets provided a sloping roof. The roof was highest where the sheets came together at the center of the hut between the two sections. A gutterlike extension just below the joining of the tin sheets caught the rain so that it could be gathered during the rainy season.

The section on the right had walls of adobe bricks that rose to a height of three feet. Above the adobe, the walls were made of cornstalks, wired together neatly. One interior wall, also of adobe and cornstalks, separated the cooking area from the bedroom. Our host explained that the cornstalks would last about three years if the rainy seasons were not too severe.

The health promoter's wife cooked on a stove made of stones, over an open wood fire, without an exhaust fan or chimney. The smoke filled the room. There were no doors of any sort in this section of the hut. The only escape route for the smoke was through the open area between the tops of the cornstalks and the tin roof, space left deliberately to vent the smoke.

Guatemalan women suffer heavily from smoke inhalation, which over a period of years causes tuberculosis. We rarely saw old women in Guatemala. Seeing the cooking room of this hut helped me understand why.

The hut's other section had wooden walls, and our host said he felt fortunate to have walls made of boards. His work with the UNICEF-sponsored project gave him a small salary, allowing him a few luxuries most peasants could not afford. This section had two rooms of equal size, one where his brothers slept, one where we were to sleep.

Our sleeping room was where the children often slept, and like them, we were to sleep on the dirt floor with a straw mat and the blankets we had brought with us, the blankets we had been instructed not to leave behind as a gift.

Our host's parents' hut had only three rooms. The largest was the kitchen, and it, too, was made of adobe and cornstalks.

"My mother is fifty-four years old," the health promoter told us proudly. She looked, by my standards, twenty years older.

Growing next to his hut were a few coffee trees, which, he said, provided enough coffee for his entire family. He also had a few chickens and ducks, and he grew a few avocados and bananas. He thought of himself as a rich and fortunate man.

The toilet was a latrine with cornstalk walls, positioned in a field of corn no more than thirty feet from the hut. The ground was unyielding, so the hole was not deep.

The washbasin was a small tin dish on a board balanced on the woodpile. There was no soap in sight.

Wood was an absolute necessity, but very expensive. Few families had land from which to harvest wood. They had to buy it. Most families burned a quetzal's worth of wood in a day, which meant that at least one-fourth of most family budgets was spent on fuel for cooking.

Everywhere in Guatemala we had seen peasants cutting, carrying, and selling stacks of firewood, in an endless cycle of earning just enough to burn just enough to eat just enough to live just another day.

Talk about Girls

We talked about family things. The health promoter's wife wanted a larger kitchen, and a new house in the village, because her husband's job with the project took most of his time and required him to be in the village instead of at home with the crops he raised on his small plot of land.

The baby was not well. He cried off and on throughout our visit. One eye was swollen, and his stomach was troubled. The baby's mother would visit with a woman in a nearby hut tomorrow to see if her neighbor had some idea that would help the child.

In the room where we were to sleep was a hen nesting with her eggs. Our hosts talked about where the hen and her nest should be taken for the night so that both would be safe from predators. Two dogs, clearly undernourished and shy, sneaked toward the kitchen and were shooed away with no sign of affection.

We asked about having dogs when food was scarce. The man said they were watchdogs. They would bark if anyone came up the path, and they did so often that night. I tried to pet the dogs, but couldn't get close to them.

We ate tortillas and beans for dinner, and had a cup of very weak coffee. The woman apologized that the beans were whole. She hadn't had time to grind them to the paste the peasants preferred. We sat on the bench in the hallway between the two sections of their hut, and the feeling among us was calm and warm.

The cooking fire flickered to glowing coals. We declined a second cup of coffee. We had been told that they rationed their supply carefully. They seldom had a second cup themselves. We tried to eat only modest portions of tortillas and beans, but our hosts kept insisting that we had not taken enough. The evening was getting damp and cool.

We retired to our room in short order and spread our mats on the dirt floor. We wrapped ourselves in our blankets and curled up for as much sleep as conditions allowed. To my surprise, I did sleep, for a time at least.

An hour or so after we retired, the two brothers, both in their teens, returned to the hut and went to their room next to ours. But not to sleep. They had come from a late church service, which they must have enjoyed thoroughly. They sang happy religious songs. They discussed the homily.

They talked bashfully, and delightedly, about the girls they had seen that night, and what adventures the future would hold if only this girl, or that girl, would smile at them in just the right way. It seemed a long time, but eventually they too slept.

Then every rooster on the mountain started crowing, and they kept crowing through most of the night.

Chuchitos for the Market

At four the next morning, or perhaps it was earlier, the grandmother kindled her cooking fire and washed her face and hands in the basin outside their hut. She moved with grace, barefoot. The soles and sides of her feet were crusted with calluses.

Her task that morning was to steam the *chuchitos* that she would carry on her head to the village. It was Sunday, market day in the village square.

Chuchitos are considered a delicacy. She had made hers the day before, with the paste that otherwise would be fried into tortillas. Into that paste she fashioned a pocket, into which she put a sauce and some small pieces of meat. Not too much meat, however. Meat was a treasure and guarded carefully. Then she formed the paste into a seamless pastry, wrapped it in fresh corn husks, and tied the husks together to keep the chuchitos neatly packaged for steaming and for the journey to the village.

In the morning, she put water in a large pot and covered the water with banana leaves. Then she put her chucoles on top of the leaves and covered them with more banana leaves. She put the pot next to the fire and let them steam.

The two young girls awoke next, just before daybreak. They washed their faces and disappeared with pans of corn that had soaked overnight in limewater. They carried the pans on their heads, without using their hands, and walked several miles to a place where, for a few cents, the corn would be ground and mixed with water to make the paste that would become the day's tortillas.

As they moved about in the early morning semi-darkness, fireworks went off in the valley. For a moment it sounded like mortar fire and I wondered if we were to be a part of another episode of violence. But it was just the way one of the churches announced that it was time to begin the journey, by foot, to the Sunday service.

Our host would normally have been up at sunrise, or earlier, but he slept late after missing the previous night's sleep. His wife entertained us and tried to comfort her sickly young son at the same time. Her daughter sat quietly next to the early morning cooking fire.

When the sun came up, we walked with her down a long, steep, rutted path to the valley floor, where a hole had been dug to capture water that ran down from the mountaintop. She filled her jar, which held perhaps four gallons, set it on her head, and with her daughter in hand, and her son in a sling on her back, she delicately carried the water back up to the hut. The journey took an hour and she made the trip three times each day.

I wasn't surprised to learn that most of the women develop serious back problems because of the loads they carry so gracefully for so many years, and because of the lack of calcium in their diet.

The cup of coffee we were given that morning was special to me. Never, I thought, had a single cup of coffee been so meaningful among strangers. My emotions were hard to contain when the grandmother sent us chuchitos for breakfast, two for each of us. She had decided each of us was to have two of her delicacies to start the day.

We had little time to visit that morning. The village would be busy with the church services and the market. We wanted to leave the area with as little commotion as possible. So we ate breakfast and said our thank-yous and goodbyes.

As we left, we offered the melon as a gift for their hospitality. They accepted it only after we agreed to take two avocados in exchange. We offered to pay for the grandmother's chucoles and were pleased when, after some gentle persuasion, they accepted the price she would have received in the village.

We met the rest of the group at the project office in the village. Everyone looked tired but somehow also refreshed and uplifted by the experience. We gathered our things quickly and put everything into our vehicles. As we did so, we noticed a man nearby, reading the morning newspapers. The headline caught our attention immediately.

The twenty disappeared peasants whom we had heard about from the man with family problems had been found.

They were all dead.

Kidnappings and assassinations
of university students and workers
are on the rise
and tortured bodies found along the highway
between Escuintla and Taxisco
have become a common sight in recent weeks.

Yet the massacre in the village of El Aguacate
against innocent peasants
can only be compared
to the Panzos massacre of earlier years.

El Grafico
Guatemala City newspaper
November 30, 1988

The army alone was not to blame—
but also a feudal and oligarchic system,
and irresponsible, corrupt civil sectors of Guatemala.

For decades the United States
favored and aided these oligarchic dictatorships,
giving lip service to democracy
but in fact pursuing its theories
of counterinsurgency and "dirty war."

The United States was really interested
only in banana republics,
in its "backyard" theory of Central America,
not in human rights.

Juan Rodil
Guatemalan Interior Minister
1988

8

A Small C

Right Direction

The twenty dead peasants we read about in Milpa were the victims of what has come to be called the El Aguacate massacre. As soon as we got back to Guatemala City on Sunday afternoon, I went to the Pan American hotel to see if the U.S. newspapers had printed anything about it, but there was no mention of it.

The group was quiet the next morning, November 28, as we drove from our hotel to our meeting with U.S. embassy officials. It was our last day in Guatemala.

We had all retired early the night before, glad to have the comfort of a hot shower and a bed with a mattress. I'd had some private time to pack, look at my notes, and wonder what it would be like to get back home just in time for the flurry of Christmas parties.

The security precautions at the office building where we met were like FUNDESA, although the armed guards weren't as numerous or as nervous. We entered a lobby decorated with wonderful works of indigenous art, which we enjoyed for a few minutes before we were guided into a small amphitheater just off the first floor.

There seemed to be tension in the group. I believe all of us felt at least some degree of disenchantment with U.S. policy in Guatemala. Some felt outright rage.

But the embassy officials who met with us were professionals, apparently accustomed to dealing with troubled, often hostile visitors from the U.S. They went through their monologues with a calm that sometimes registered as boredom.

One of the men worked with the embassy's public information program. The other was with the AID effort. I guessed them both to be in their thirties. They were competent looking, dressed in suits and ties, though they quickly shed their coats and projected a more relaxed image.

We were not allowed to take pictures or use our tape recorders, and later Mary asked me not to use their names in this book. The meeting was supposed to be "off the record," whatever that means.

They began defensively, clearly expecting the meeting to be difficult. They seemed to want to neutralize as much of our outrage as they could.

The AID man spoke about the improvements in Guatemala since 1969, a time when he said there had been "no hope" for Guatemala ever seeing any form of democratic process. By 1983, the situation had improved to the point where there was a consensus that there would never again be a dictatorship in Guatemala, of the left or the right. He reminded us that there were a lot of problems in Boston and Alabama, too. Sure, there was more violence in Guatemala; but the country was on the move, he said, "in the right direction."

Human Rights

Someone asked the officials to give their impression of the human rights situation, especially since the coup attempt of May 11, 1988. The officials seemed surprised that they had been interrupted so early in their patter.

"There is a problem, but less than in past years," one said. Human rights violations now were not directed by the government, as they had been in the regimes of Lucas Garcia or Rios Montt. Today's violence was the result of extremists on both the left and right. Violence was "outside the intentions of the government."

In fact, he said, many victims of the violence were members of the government, although that was becoming less common. President Cerezo had recently remarked, with officers of the Guatemala army seated all around him, that "I'm only here today because these guys were such rotten shots."

We asked about yesterday's headline—the twenty bodies that had been found so close to where we had slept two nights before.

They had been killed, one of the officials said, by "a demoralized guerrilla force taking vengeance." Since the coup attempt it had become difficult to distinguish between violence that was a result of a growing criminal trend and violence that was a result of politics.

The other official said the embassy got its information on human rights violations by analyzing press reports and police data sheets. The problem, he said, was partly a matter of definitions. A violent political act was one in which political motivation could not be ruled out, but motivation was sometimes difficult to interpret. The U.S. embassy's numbers on human rights abuses were, therefore, usually lower than those of Americas Watch, as were the numbers generated by the Guatemalan government.

Guatemala, he said, "has no effective criminal justice system. It's still vigilante style." Things were improving, however.

To illustrate the improvement, he told us about a judge who had been murdered recently. Once, the incident would have been blown up into an enormous scandal, with lots of accusations about political motivation and extremists and so on. But because of the training the U.S. has provided in investigatory technique, the perpetrator was found to be the judge's son, who had killed his father in a family dispute.

"That defused a big deal," he said.

As a further illustration, he said that a prominent U.S. citizen had been shot recently, and was in a coma. The incident would normally have been given lots of press attention, creating many stories about human rights abuses. But the fact was that the U.S. citizen was shot when his own gun dropped.

I wondered if these were more "shoeless millionaire bus driver" stories.

Programs

Someone asked the AID representative to describe some of the AID programs and tell us how much money actually reached the peasants.

He said AID had many programs in Guatemala, and that U.S. aid was used, in large part, to help Guatemala's balance of payments. He said the country had made progress since 1986. The key to further progress was to bring the economically disastrous civil war to an end. He spoke in the calm monotone of an accountant going over a tax return, and he did not elaborate.

He did not say how peace could be restored within the context of low-intensity conflict and the government's refusal to negotiate with the guerrillas. He did not say how peace could be restored without reasonable compliance with the Esquipulas II agreement, nor did he say how the Cerezo government could declare that there was no need for dialogue with the guerrillas because the guerrillas did not exist.

He moved instead to the subject of export crops and AID agricultural projects. He said a strawberry initiative was working well; the problem now was how to replicate it in quantity. The goal was to improve production for export, and to diversify Guatemalan agriculture.

He did not discuss the impact of the export orientation on either the peasants or the country's foreign debt.

Another AID goal was to improve the mortality rate among children. Forty percent died before age five, he said, using a number lower than we were used to hearing. AID sponsored several immunization and oral-rehydration projects.

Simply surviving wasn't enough, however, he said. The people "gotta have something to live for."

That led him to a comment on education. Some eight hundred bilingual schools in the highlands received AID support. Some sixty-four thousand children attended these schools. And the girls were staying in these schools, which was something new and important.

Initially, the U.S. had paid half the cost of these schools. Now

Guatemala paid three-quarters of the cost. Parents paid for their children's uniforms.

Training teachers was the biggest challenge, he said. They had to be fluent in both Spanish and one of the indigenous languages; and they had to be sensitive to the traditions and the human difficulties of the country.

Before Guatemala could move forward on matters like health and education, he said, the country had to "create a stronger tax base" and "get government more involved."

I thought about Bendfelt at FUNDESA, who thought the government was already too involved. Bendfelt, however, represented an elite, to whom taxes were the equivalent of socialism.

Democracy

Someone asked what criteria the embassy used to define democracy or apply it to the Guatemalan culture.

The AID representative said that without a promising future, democracy meant nothing. With a hopeless present, democracy meant nothing. The issue was "ballots, not bullets," he said.

The presence of democracy was tested in Guatemala by two things. First, the violence had to disappear. Second, the "little guy" had to be "plugged into economic opportunity."

When he talked about the little guy and the need for peace, I at last felt a bond with him, as, I believe, did others in the group. The man himself seemed to show through the professional veneer. What he had said about democracy didn't sound like the administration line; it sounded like the statement of an individual who cared. It sounded like truth. He emphasized that the ballot box was working.

In April 1988, Guatemala had held municipal elections, in which the Christian Democratic Party did well, frustrating the efforts of those who were inclined to keep the "little guy" out.

One member of our group wasn't satisfied with the response, however. He said a recent U.S. newspaper article had quoted President Cerezo as saying he would not investigate past crimes against human rights. The questioner wanted to know if that sounded like democracy and why more guns were needed in Guatemala if democracy was making progress.

The mood became somber. The AID representative seemed to be trying to control his emotions.

"You can't compare U.S. to Guatemalan democracy," he said. In the U.S. Civil War and the Indian wars, amnesties were declared immediately after the hostilities ceased. The precedent for amnesty was present even in U.S. history. The same precedent had been set in Brazil, although Argentina had been a different case.

Compromises are made, he said. "Guatemalans are willing to accept such compromises to make some progress, such as the army cleaning itself up."

Amazing They Trust Us

The public-information man stepped in at this point, speaking in a friendlier tone. There "seems to be real structural change" going on in Guatemala, he said.

He used that comment to preface his assertion that the recent sale of M-16s was strictly commercial. The U.S. government's involvement was limited to approving a license for the sale. I felt he was minimizing, but his calmness saved the meeting from degenerating into an argument.

Only about $10 million out of $150 million in U.S. aid was military, he said, and that $10 million was nonlethal. As far as the M-16s were concerned, Guatemala was going to buy them anyway.

It occurred to me that "nonlethal military aid" was a contradiction in terms.

"The army is fighting a war. The guerrillas are getting their guns from Cuba and Nicaragua." Their weapons, he said, were U.S. M-16s from the Vietnam conflict, smuggled into Guatemala over the Mexican border.

Only a thousand out of ten thousand guerrillas were hard core Marxist-Leninists, the AID representative said, but even these radicals could be protected under the amnesty provisions.

The discussion was drifting. I found the AID representative's emotionalism troubling, as was the return to party-line rhetoric after a tender moment.

Someone asked about credibility, suggesting that it was difficult to trust the U.S. government anymore, especially considering the CIA's role in the 1954 coup that overthrew President Jacobo Arbenz Guzman. Curiously, the question seemed to refresh the officials, and they seemed to relax.

"Could it happen again?" the public-information officer asked rhetorically.

The harbor in Nicaragua had been mined by the U.S., he said. It was true that there was reason for cynicism. Reporters were cynical. There was the Freedom of Information Act. There was Vietnam. There were "high moral leakers." And all of that "makes my job tougher sometimes.

"So, the U.S. government can't get away with that stuff," he said. The U.S. wasn't having much success with Noriega in Panama, he said. We could be more trusting of our government simply because there was so much more suspicion.

Another good question, the AID representative said, was, "How can Guatemala trust us? Sometimes I wonder. Indeed, we've pulled off a lot of little stunts around here."

His sudden moment of candor surprised me again.

"Yet they trust in the U.S. and democracy. It's amazing they trust us as well as they do."

The public-information officer said, "We really don't speak with one voice in foreign policy anymore. We open and close spigots. Our partners can't depend on the U.S. — Americas Watch wants aid cut off." It would be difficult to find comfort in a relationship with the U.S. One politician would say one thing; another politician would say something else. One day money would be forthcoming; the next day it wouldn't be. Groups advocated one thing or another. Policy shifted. Tactics changed.

The U.S. Congress had passed a law, he said—if there was a coup, the U.S. would stop its aid.

"There's some comfort in checks and balances."

A World of Dreams

Another person asked about land reform, noting that there wasn't much land for the "little people."

"Land distribution is an enormous problem," the AID representative said. "There probably isn't enough land for everybody."

Some commercial farms had worked well, but there weren't enough of them to affect the whole population. And the land problem was connected to the terrain itself.

"The lowlands belong to people," he said, emphasizing the word "belong," as though it were sacred — a part of the religion of private property.

"Highland Indians don't want to go to the coast. Yet the highlands are overpopulated."

The answer, if there was any, might be in education, or perhaps in diversification of the economy.

"Expropriatory land reform has never worked anywhere," he said. No one questioned him on this, but I thought back to the reform period under presidents Arevalo and Arbenz, whose expropriatory land reform was so successful that it served as a guide in the development of President Kennedy's Alliance for Progress program.

"As to the bishops' letter" on land reform, he said, "I don't pay a lot of attention. They live in a world of dreams. Don't confuse the letter with the possible. It's not real, not solutions. Bishops are not economists."

A Small C

Someone changed the subject, and I was grateful for it. The meeting had become extremely tense again. The question was about the government's education and health budget, which had been cut recently, and about why Rigoberta Menchu and others in the peasant community had been excluded from the national dialogue.

The budget for health and education had not been cut, the

official said. The problem was the delivery system. The majority of the budget was consumed by the bureaucracy. The embassy wanted the government budget to expand, but with the qualification that private systems be used to deliver the actual services.

It's important to "see Guatemala as a motion picture, not a snapshot," one of them said. The motion picture would show progress. The snapshot would cause dismay.

They said nothing about the national dialogue.

I asked them to help me understand their definition of communism. They had said that their AID projects in agriculture were of a communal nature.

In the Midwest, I said, and probably throughout the United States, there were many agricultural cooperatives. When, in their opinion, did something stop being a cooperative and start being communism?

They paused for a short time. Then one said that some of the Indian land ownership was communal. He seemed to be talking while he tried to think of an answer. Then he surprised me by saying, "No one has a problem with communism with a small C. You can't title land to the country as a whole."

AID money is bilateral, he said, and intended for maximum private sector delivery, not intended for expanding a government bureaucracy. I had the sense that he was scrambling for a way to explain the concept of small C communism.

"Padre Giron is a friend of mine," he blurted out.

I wasn't sure what he was getting at in these disconnected comments, but I was sure that political theory was a spectrum of grays, rather than a polarization of black and white.

Vigilante Era

Someone asked about the popular movement and its leadership, which had been virtually wiped out in the 1980s. What was the embassy perspective on where the movement was now?

The officials said that the popular movement had been bolstered by the training its leaders had received at Loyola, in New Orleans, with U.S. support. They admitted that many of the leaders of popular organizations had been murdered in the violence.

With that they left the question unanswered, and the meeting began to deteriorate again. People shuffled in their seats and looked around to see if anyone else wanted to ask a question.

Someone asked about U.S. involvement in the violence of the 1980s, and the officials' response danced around the question. They said Europe stayed away from Central American affairs during the 1980s, even though there were Christian Democrats in Europe. But that was changing; Europe was becoming more involved. They hadn't been asked about Europe.

Someone asked if export agriculture was the wrong strategy. "No farmer is stupid," they said. "They don't abandon corn and beans to grow sugar and starve. They gain up to five percent in income."

The U.S. Drug Omnibus law had killed two shipments of Guatemalan strawberries because of delays in inspection, he said. I wasn't sure how that connected with the question, which was about starving people.

Someone asked about the new strategy of stabilization.

The military was now receiving training in human rights, they said, although it "had been an army of occupation." The answers were getting shorter.

Another question dealt with the risk people took on when they got involved in reform programs. The officials admitted that in Guatemala those who wanted to effect change always ran a risk. "Threats are a way of life" in Guatemala. In the States, one said, "We say 'stuff it.' But here it might be serious." Journalists received threats constantly. People were reminded that "we know where you live." But things were changing.

To conclude, one official said it was important for us to remember that it "took a while to get out of the U.S. vigilante era." All too often, they said, people were simply looking for a "high platform to damn the world."

The meeting was over. So was my sabbatical. I was tired.

As we drove back to the Colonial Hotel, I realized again that Guatemala was polarized in every way possible—economically, one was either rich or poor; socially, one was either Indian or ladino; politically, one was an advocate of either the private or the public sector; theologically, one was either conservative or progressive. As a visitor, and since that time as a student of the country, I felt pulled toward one extreme or the other while I searched, without much success, for people and ideas in the middle. Worse, all the evidence suggested that the extremes were moving further apart and the voids in the middle were becoming larger.

The embassy officials had acted as though they wanted to shoo us away as they would shoo away pestering children, or as our host in the mountains shooed away his watchdogs. Padre Tomas's analogy of the fly stinging the conscience of the elephant came back to me.

I had hoped the embassy officials would help fill the voids in the middle somewhat, but they didn't, except for volunteering that there was such a thing as communism with a small C. Otherwise they made me feel that they were among the agents of polarization.

They acted as if they had some kind of master plan that would solve everything someday. Yet all the facts suggested that was not the case. They acted as if they were on top of things. Yet they talked about the divergent pressures within our government and how difficult it was for other countries to trust us.

I came away feeling strongly that U.S. citizens—the many plain, unbiased, average, decent people who are the real soul of our country—were desperately needed to monitor our government's actions, and that abdication of that responsibility to Washington and to embassies like that in Guatemala City was frightfully dangerous.

Throughout the trip, I felt torn between cynicism and naivete. I decided consciously that if I erred, it would be on the side of naivete. In that I was sure I would receive a great deal of correction. In cynicism, however, I feared I might simply blend in with those who acted as if they were on top of things. Cynicism, I came to feel, was also frightfully dangerous. I could not see how it would make anything better.

I remembered that Padre Tomas had said the situation was crazy. Maria Emilia Garcia and the health promoter simply stared through their pain and fatigue. Father John didn't want to talk about it. Padre Andres was resigned to whatever might happen. But all five were determined, and all five would stay in my memory and prevent me from denying those things that can't be neatly understood. They would go on, I was certain, and do the best they could for as long as they could.

Early the next morning we left Guatemala City. I may never return, and yet there will never be a distance separating my heart from the beauty of the country or the miraculous spirit of its enduring people.

———————

Systems that allow the exploitation of man by man
should not be permitted,
nor should corruption
or situations in which some have too much
while others, through no fault of their own,
lack everything.

Let there be no families that are destroyed,
separated and without sufficient help;
let there be no one without the protection of the law,
which is to protect all without distinction.

Force should never prevail over truth and law,
nor economic and political systems
over the dignity of man.

Pope John Paul II
Mexico, 1979

———————

There is a crime here
that goes beyond denunciation.

There is a sorrow here
that weeping cannot symbolize.

There is a failure here
that topples all our success . . .
and in the eyes of the hungry
there is a growing wrath.

In the souls of the people
the grapes of wrath are filling
and growing heavy,
growing heavy for the vintage.

John Steinbeck
The Grapes of Wrath

Conclusion

A Basic Choice

I don't know how hard my heart had been before I went to Guatemala, but I could feel it changing almost minute by minute while I was there. Since then, hardness of heart has been very much on my mind.

At times, we met with people in whom I sensed little compassion. They denied the existence of suffering, violence, and injustice. I felt they were trying to sell me something.

But during the rest of the trip, in lesson after painful lesson, the softening process was at work, and it has continued during the year of study, conversation, and thought that went into the writing of this book.

At its core, Guatemala and perhaps all of Central America is an issue of heart, not of politics or ideology or even theology; not of economics or national security or ecology or culture. These things are all involved, but at the center is the matter of individual hearts.

A hardened heart comes from distance and denial, and from living in the rat race, and maybe from an insecurity that someone higher up might not be pleased if a flaw is noticed or a suggestion is made.

A softened heart requires courage, and stirs compassion. Compassion brings with it grieving and conversion.

In Guatemala, I learned the real meaning of adventure, and of being a Christian. I learned again not to be self-righteous lest someone remind me of my own problems, as Baetz reminded us about the pornography that comes to Guatemala from the U.S.

I saw things I'll never forget: the omnipresent military patrols, the slums, the crowded streets and parks, the smog, the headlines that Sunday morning after the El Aguacate massacre. I saw a beautiful country and beautiful people. A country deteriorating. A people suffering. Policies that don't work.

Every Father's Day I will remember the orphans marching, posting their lonely cards on Guatemala City walls: "Father, where are you?" "Father, come home, we miss you." "Father, we pray you are safe. We love you."

Volcanoes will have a new meaning too. So will campfires: during the worst of the violence, the dead were stacked so high that people began to refer to them as *leña*, which means firewood.

Things *have* changed in Guatemala. They're worse—more dangerous to us, to our security, to our souls. The people are poorer, their scars deeper and more painful. The population is larger, younger, better organized, and more aware. Women are more involved—active and angry. The economy is awful. The ecology is deteriorating. The fundamental problems of starvation and injustice are increasing.

What is not new is the tenacious way the comfortable in both Guatemala and the U.S. cling to myths: the myth that the peasants are not truly poor because the nonmonetary economy compensates them; the myth that Guatemala is not our problem in the U.S.; the myth that violence is necessary in Guatemala and that it is acceptable because they are only killing demons; the myth that guns solve problems; the myth that Guatemalans are inferior; the myth that religion and reality need to be kept separate.

The acceptance of myth is a barrier between self and the grieving that's necessary for conversion, a barrier to personal exodus, a barrier to the answer to each individual's First Commandment question: "Who is your God?"

I didn't believe much in miracles before I went to Guatemala. I do now. The strength of the people there, their love and will to endure, their support of each other—those are miracles. The miracle of life. The miracle of sharing.

I felt little connection between history and my own life before.

Now I feel everyone is an historical person, everyone has an historical moment.

Everyone has a choice, too, about what is conditional and what is unconditional. If the use of property is unconditional, injustice and violence can result, as they have in Guatemala. If love is unconditional, who knows what might result.

Our Living Room

There's a supermarket a few miles away from my home. It's average in size, which means that it offers a consumer over twenty thousand items. When I walk through its aisles now I think about how many things we have in our supermarkets, department stores, shopping malls, and other outlets. Most U.S. consumers have abundant choices, and convenience, and affordable prices. We can buy coffee, beef, bananas, and sugar, for example, for a few cents or a few dollars per pound.

The first cup of coffee in the morning is a special treat for me. But now it combines with a reflection on land, owned by a few, that is dedicated to exporting the coffee, sugar, and beef that I can buy for a few cents or a few dollars a pound. I realize now that peasants have been pushed off that land, and earn perhaps a dollar a day to harvest those export crops. And a dollar a day is not enough to sustain them.

I think about Guatemala's foreign debt, which keeps growing, and how Guatemala responds, and is urged to respond, by emphasizing export crops even more. So more peasants are pushed off more land.

The foreign debt and those who profit from the exports have voracious appetites. Forests become victims, too, as trees come down so that more cattle may graze and more crops may grow. Half the forests Central America had in 1950 are gone.

The debt consumes much of the foreign aid we provide—that and military expenses. I used to think of the U.S. as a generous nation until I studied our foreign aid. The reality is that we aren't very generous at all. At least sixteen other countries give a greater percentage of their gross domestic product. Israel and Egypt get half our aid. Take out that half, and our aid for servicing foreign debt—which channels U.S. taxpayers' money to U.S. bankers—and our military assistance, and what's left isn't very much.

That morning cup of coffee brings reflections, too, on military aid, and on the use of guns. I used to believe that such aid had something to do with safeguarding democracy and economic development. But it's just not that simple. The only simple reality is that guns kill, and fascist violence is as bad as any other violence. The key question is: democracy and development for whom? For the poor, or for just a few?

Democracy is superior to any other system, even with its imperfections. But democracy doesn't exist simply because political rhetoric declares that it exists, nor does it exist simply because an election is held. The very presence of all the guns is testimony to the lack of democracy, a signal that something is very wrong.

We have to ask about pluralism and participation. We have to ask about the tolerance for differing points of view. We have to ask whether the poor would vote to stay poor, whether the illiterate would vote to stay illiterate, and whether the landless would vote for politicians who extend the polarization and injustice of the country.

Our military aid should trouble our souls, and so should this new strategy called low-intensity conflict. These things go beyond ideology, rhetoric and labels. They are moral matters, and matters for the conscience. They sustain injustice. They continue because of hardened hearts and the deadly D's—distancing and denial.

There are, certainly, opportunists ready to exploit circumstances, and they must be kept in check. The critical issue, however, is those circumstances—the fundamental problems, the suffering and the injustice. If we work on the fundamentals, the exploiters have less to exploit.

But in my living room in Minneapolis with my morning cup of coffee, it's easier to think about labels and East-West ideological conflict. The labels are simple and convenient; they allow me distance, and support my denial. The ideologies are cerebral; they allow me to avoid the grief of being close to suffering people.

I look around my living room, however, and think how awful it would be if someone were killed or tortured in one of its corners, or if a baby starved to death there. I think it would be even more awful if there were a connection between that killing or that baby's starvation and my morning cup of coffee.

Friends, there is such a connection. This earth is *our* living room. We must study its corners more carefully because they are filling with suffering and angry people.

Heavenly Father,
we bow our heads
and thank You for Your love.

Accept our thanks
for the peace that yields this day
and the shared faith
that makes its continuance likely.

Make us strong to do Your work,
willing to heed and hear Your will,
and write on our hearts these words:

"Use power to help people."

For we are given power
not to advance our own purposes,
nor to make a great show in the world,
nor a name.

There is but one just use of power,
and it is to serve people.

Help us remember, Lord. Amen.

President George Bush
Inaugural Address
January 20, 1989

Appendix A

History and Status

Our first meeting in Guatemala was with our guides, who provided us with an overview of the country's history and current situation. What follows is a condensation of the information provided in that session.

Guatemala was conquered by Spain in 1524, but the word "conquered" is misleading. Horses were not native to the Americas, and the horses the Spaniards rode struck fear into the hearts of the Indians. So a handful of Spanish soldiers, together with their horses and an army of Mexican mercenaries, were able to take control of a region in which the Indian tribes were already divided.

Twenty-three indigenous languages are still spoken in Guatemala. Indigenous costume is worn throughout the country. The patterns are passed down through the generations, and each pattern represents a specific tribe.

One by-product of the attacks on indigenous culture has been the creation of common languages—Spanish and four main Indian languages. These common languages have made for greater unity among the Indian people, who make up roughly half the population.

The Spanish were not interested in colonizing Guatemala. Their purpose was simply to get out as much wealth as possible as quickly as possible and get it back to Europe. Such economic and political structures as were established were to facilitate that purpose, and these structures stayed in place after Guatemala achieved its independence in 1821.

Rufino Barrios

Guatemala's major wealth in the early 1800s was in the production of export crops, especially sugar. The country was dominated by the Con-

179

servatives, who controlled everything in society and did so until late in the century, when the Liberals took power for a short time.

In 1871, a Liberal president, Justo Rufino Barrios, set out to make the economy more progressive, and to do this the government expropriated communal lands as well as land owned by the Catholic Church. The Liberal philosophy advocated greater distance between the Church and government.

In confiscating Church lands and depriving the Church of a major, though indirect, role in government affairs, the Barrios administration interrupted a centuries-old alliance between the leaders of society and the leaders of the Church.

With the expropriated land, Rufino Barrios developed a coffee trade, and he recruited Germans to help this emerging segment of the country's agriculture. The Germans and the coffee growers became a second tier of the country's oligarchy, less feudal than the sugar growers, and more inclined to pay workers so that they could purchase goods and keep the economy active.

The cultivation of coffee reinforced Guatemala's dependence on export trade, and that reinforced the consolidation of land in the hands of a few.

In 1876, Ruffino Barrios attempted to unify Central America under Guatemalan leadership. Meetings were held in Guatemala City, but the delegates argued endlessly over details. By 1885, Rufino Barrios's patience with the unification project was at an end. He issued an ultimatum, in which he was supported only by Honduras. To note its displeasure with his unification scheme, the United States sent warships to threaten Barrios.

Barrios invaded El Salvador anyway, but a sniper's bullet ended his life, and thus ended one of the few attempts to unite the tiny countries of Central America.

Shortly after Barrios's death, the United Fruit Company came to Guatemala. It soon became the dominant force, not only in agriculture, but in all economic and political affairs. The United Fruit Company continued to control the country until the 1950s.

In the post-Barrios years, Guatemala was governed by a series of dictators friendly to the interests of the United States and generally controlled by the U.S. companies operating in Guatemala.

Arevalo and Arbenz

The last of those dictators was Jorge Ubico, who ruled from 1931 until 1944. During this period, as the country's economy continued to grow, a small middle class began to emerge. This middle-class element became dissatisfied with Ubico's leadership, and aided by the country's military, it overthrew the dictator.

What followed was a decade of nominal reform, which began with the presidency of Juan Jose Arevalo. Arevalo introduced a minimum-wage program, reduced the work week, and allowed unions and strikes. But on the fundamental question of land reform, Arevalo's initiatives were moderate, and even then they were strongly resisted by the oligarchy.

As Guatemala became more and more involved with the export of sugar and coffee, the peasants were moved off the land. They had to depend on smaller plots of lower-quality ground for the staples they needed. They were pushed off the fertile plains near the Pacific Ocean and moved into the mountains to grow their crops on steep slopes with marginal soil.

Throughout Guatemala's history, land has been the central concern of the people and the core of the nation's economic problems. The indigenous people feel a strong spiritual attachment to the land, and especially to the corn that can be grown on it.

As the population grew, it exacerbated the problem. The Indian population needed more land to feed itself; the oligarchs needed more land to increase the return on their investment in export crops.

In 1950, Jacobo Arbenz Guzman succeeded Arevalo. Arbenz's answer to Guatemala's economic problems was to increase wages so that people could buy goods. Industries could then be developed to manufacture those goods.

The bulk of Guatemala's population, however, was involved in subsistence farming. This meant that the only way to create purchasing power was to set up a structure that allowed the peasants to feed themselves and still have something left over to sell for cash, which they in turn would spend on the country's manufactured goods.

That meant land reform. The reform Arbenz proposed was to be accomplished by expropriating idle lands. Owners would be compensated for the value they had claimed for the land when they paid their real estate taxes. The expropriated land would be divided into plots large enough to sustain a peasant family and allow a surplus.

The landowners, however, would have none of this scenario. Neither would the United Fruit Company, nor would the United States. Arbenz was overthrown by the U.S. in 1954, through the efforts of its new geopolitical weapon, the CIA.

Arbenz had been a constitutionally elected president. He had come to power in a free and fair election, symbolic of the democracy the U.S. prizes. The 1954 coup is one of the milestone events in the relationship of the United States and Central America. Democracy was subverted for the sake of economic privilege.

The 1960s

Following the 1954 coup, Guatemala was ruled by a series of military governments. Wealth became even more concentrated, and repression became a constant in the lives of the poor.

In the late 1950s and in the 1960s, dissatisfaction with the military government, and with the concentration of wealth, coalesced into an armed opposition—the guerrilla movement.

Also during the 1960s, many populist groups sprang up, and their activities were nourished by the increasingly progressive orientation of the Catholic Church.

"Base Christian communities," a term we were told was not safe to use in Guatemala, became numerous and active, especially in the highlands. Peasant organizations grew. Unions, which had been destroyed and outlawed following the 1954 coup, began to appear again.

The health promoters movement began in the '60s. Its primary work was helping people cure and prevent illness, but it went a step further. As our guide Mary described it, "A peasant boy might cut his foot, and the promoter would ask the mother why the foot was cut.

"She would say, 'Because the boy had no shoes.' The promoter would ask why the boy had no shoes. She would say he has no shoes because the family cannot afford to buy them.

"The promoter would ask why the family cannot afford to buy them. She would say because their land is not big enough to grow crops to feed the family and have anything left over to sell for money to buy the shoes. And the promoter would ask why isn't their plot of land big enough.

"Gradually she would realize that the ownership of land in her area, which was concentrated in the hands of a few, had something directly to do with the cut on the foot of her son.

"She would tell her neighbor what she learned. Her neighbor would pass it on."

The health promoters' efforts coordinated naturally with the work of the progressive clergy and of other populist groups. Peasants often met together in base Christian communities to discuss the causes of their poverty and to ask themselves what they might do about it. The catechists who led the meetings of the base Christian communities became the primary targets of the counterinsurgency.

Guerrilla Gettysburg

In the 1970s, popular support for political alternatives was strong. The Christian Democratic Party seemed ready to make useful reforms and certain to win the 1974 presidential election. But immediately after the votes were cast, the electronic media went dead throughout the country. Nothing was heard for several days. When broadcasting resumed, the military candidate was declared the winner.

The guerrilla movement received a powerful impetus.

"People took to the hills with guns," Mary told us. "They said, 'That's the only way we can change this government. We tried due electoral process. It didn't work.' "

By the late 1970s, violence was more intense than it had been during the previous decade. In the cities, union and student leaders were disappeared, killed, or tortured. Journalists, middle-class people, doctors, anyone who was suspected of supporting structural change became a target. In the rural areas, the targets were teachers, populist leaders, health promoters, and especially catechists. From 1978 on, death-squad activities were in full swing.

Still the guerrilla movement grew. By 1981, the guerrillas controlled between one-third and one-half the country. They controlled the transportation corridor that ran from Huehuetenango past Lake Atitlan to the capital city.

Some people believe that had the guerillas been willing to make the attempt, they could have conquered the country.

They're Just Indians

In March 1982, an evangelical Protestant, General Efraim Rios Montt, came to power in yet another coup. Under his leadership, counterinsurgency strategy became more sophisticated.

Rios Montt eliminated some of the corruption within the military, and as the military became more efficient, it focused more effectively on the task of eliminating the guerillas. An even more violent period began, perhaps the most violent in the country's long history of terror.

The Rios Montt antiguerrilla program contained elements conceived of and taught by the U.S. military based on its experience in Vietnam. Entire villages were destroyed. The army itself acknowledges the destruction of 440 villages. Massacres were common.

In the late '70s and early '80s, the repression was concentrated in Guatemala City. It focused primarily on student and labor organizations.

The urban repression diminished somewhat under Rios Montt, but in its place came massive violence in the countryside.

Tom, our escort from Minneapolis, said, "You'll hear people from the city say that when Rios Montt came to power the repression ended. What they're really saying is that it was reduced here in the city, but not in the countryside.

"The evangelical fervor was important because there was a whole justification behind the repression—that the Indian people were not Christians.

"So there was a lot of preaching going on about 'It's okay to kill them. They're just Indians. They're just communists.'"

Over a hundred thousand people were killed during the violence of the early 1980s. Perhaps five thousand of these were armed guerrillas. At least forty thousand other people disappeared.

Amnesty

By the time Rios Montt was overthrown in 1983, the worst of the violence was over. His successor, General Oscar Mejia Victores, began a process of reconstruction, using the "model village" to concentrate people into locations where they could be controlled more easily.

By 1984, the country was in large part pacified but in a serious economic condition. Years of supporting a large, corrupt, and inefficient military had taken their toll, as had high oil prices and low prices for Guatemala's exports.

Most international aid had been cut off. This included aid from the U.S., which was suspended because of human rights violations.

To bolster the economy and keep the counterinsurgency program alive, the power structure took several steps. A new constitution was written. Elections were held in 1985, and a Christian Democrat, Vinicio Cerezo, was elected president in what most people considered fair elections for those parties that were allowed to run.

The main question at the time was whether that event marked a change in the fundamental power structure of the country, or whether the election was simply a cosmetic that allowed Guatemala to obtain foreign aid and loans.

Shortly before the military turned over the presidency to Vinicio Cerezo, however, it passed the Amnesty Decree, stating that no one could be prosecuted for any political or military crimes committed since March 1982—in other words, since Rios Montt came to power.

U.S. Role

Mary told us that the U.S. had an indirect role in the counterinsurgency. "As early as the mid-'70s, Israel was becoming a major arms supplier for Guatemala, and so when Carter cut off military aid and weapons sales in 1979, Israel was already in place as the primary arms supplier and trainer.

"A lot of training also took place in South Africa and in Taiwan. And so the U.S. role was not direct, especially not in the way you see it, for example, in El Salvador, where the U.S. is giving half the country's budget, and where our military trainers are legal."

Tom added that he had asked an authority on Guatemala, Jean-Marie Simon, about the U.S. role and had been told that that role was minimal for the simple reason that it wasn't needed.

"The U.S. had done such a good job in the 1960s," he said, "when the Green Berets were here training the Guatemalan military in counterinsurgency tactics—really the first time they had done that in Latin America—that there was no need to do here what they are currently doing in El Salvador and to some extent in Honduras."

The Guatemalan counterinsurgency effort was sophisticated. Israeli computers were used to monitor energy consumption. Guerrilla safe houses could be detected through their late-night consumption of electrical power for printing presses and lights.

The Guatemalan military had also received from Israel the technology it needed to manufacture its own ammunition.

Temporary Partnership

Cerezo was inaugurated in January 1986. Mary characterized the period this way: "The far left, the guerrilla insurgents, and the far right, the feudal far right, for want of a better term, were pretty much marginalized from the political scene. Cerezo had a little room to move in, and there was some room for popular organizations again, and they did start to organize.

"The military at that point was pretty much behind Cerezo in terms of democratization and the improvement of the country's image."

Cerezo traveled abroad, announcing that democracy had come to Guatemala and seeking international aid.

Human rights violations declined early in his administration, although they increased again in late 1987, and they had increased further in the six months before I visited Guatemala.

Mary said she saw Cerezo as a junior partner to the military and the business elite during his first two years. Then the partnership began to fall apart. His role in the Esquipulas Central American peace agreement antagonized the Guatemalan military, but even worse for the partnership was the short dialogue between the government and the guerrillas in Madrid in October 1987. That meeting broke up quickly without accomplishing much other than antagonizing the Guatemalan military.

The partnership with the business elite deteriorated when Cerezo introduced several tax initiatives, one of which was designed to improve the tax-collection system. And the popular sector became unhappy when Cerezo proposed a forty percent increase in electricity rates.

In January 1988, Guatemala experienced the largest protest demonstrations it had seen since 1980. They were organized by Popular and Labor Action Unity. These demonstrations led to a meeting with the government and an agreement, signed in March.

The March accord was comprehensive. Electricity rates were not to be increased the proposed forty percent, but scaled upward, with heavy users receiving larger increases. The prices of basic items were to be placed under a system of controls. Private-sector employees were to receive a fifty quetzales (about fifteen dollars) a month increase.

The accord also called for the formation of an investigatory commission on human rights abuses, and the Campesino Unity Committee was officially recognized.

In April, members of the Unified Guatemalan Opposition, a political opposition group outside the country, sent a delegation to Guatemala to see if the situation had changed. Esquipulas II, the second set of peace accords signed by the presidents of the Central American countries, provided that opposition representatives would be allowed to travel about the country to review conditions and verify their improvement. Exiles and refugees were to be free to return without harm.

So the opposition group sent four delegates, including Rigoberta Menchu, of the newly recognized Campesino Unity Committee. She and one other delegate were arrested at the airport, detained for the day, then released when protests began to build.

This outraged the military, because it considered Menchu and the others members of the armed opposition. The civilian-military partnership collapsed, and there was a coup attempt on May 11.

Coups and coup attempts are frequent occurrences in Guatemalan history. What was surprising about this attempt was that it was directed against Cerezo, a civilian who was effectively doing the one thing the country desperately needed done—getting foreign aid.

Although the coup did not topple the government, it was successful in other ways. The minister of the interior was replaced. The March accord was not implemented. Prices were allowed to increase. No wage increases were forthcoming.

Political violence increased. Union leaders were killed. Others were threatened. Several members of university student organizations were killed, tortured, or forced to leave the country.

At the time I was in Guatemala, Mary described the situation as "fairly tense. The very far right seems to be pacified a little bit by the fact that the government has done many of the things that it wanted, but it continues to speak of coups. There have been rumors. It continues to be a threat."

Populist organizations were growing, and they continued to organize and demonstrate. The Christian Democratic Party was losing support from all sides and becoming defensive.

The armed opposition was also getting stronger, although it was not nearly as strong as it had been in 1981.

With this, our briefing was over, and we prepared for the meetings discussed in this book.

Update

Since my trip to Guatemala, the violations of human rights have increased. Some believe that the increase is intended to embarrass Cerezo's Christian Democratic Party and ease the way for a more conservative candidate. Others believe Cerezo will not complete his term. Another coup attempt failed in May 1989.

International coffee prices have fallen, adding more problems to the troubled economy. In July 1989, 100-pound bags of Central American coffee sold for $77, one-third of their 1986 level. Each $1 drop costs Guatemala $4 million in earnings.

The foreign debt keeps climbing. The ecology keeps deteriorating— Central America has half the forest land it had in 1950.

Early in 1989, the country experienced the largest worker strike since 1980. Over fifty thousand plantation workers demanded higher wages and better conditions. The strike was unsuccessful. Later in the year, the country's school system was paralyzed by a teachers' strike, which also ended without major gains for the strikers. Since the strikes, union and student leaders have been killed, tortured, and disappeared.

U.S. aid continues to flow into Guatemala.

Press attention in the U.S. remains focused elsewhere in Central America—on Nicaragua, Panama, and El Salvador. The Guatemalan press, however, receives its share of violent attention—bombings, threats, beatings.

Guatemala's justice system has yet to prosecute any official for human rights crimes. Most cases are simply dismissed for lack of evidence. Sometimes judge and attorney become victims of violence as well.

Members of the clergy continue to be persecuted—forced into exile, kidnapped, tortured, and disappeared. In the last decade, seventeen priests and sisters, three from the U.S., were killed or disappeared.

The guerrilla war has increased. Casualties in the Guatemalan military are reported as heavy. The morale among lower-level officers is reported to be poor because of the casualties and lack of support. The government continues to deny the war and refuses to acknowledge the guerrillas as a threat or a legitimate party to Esquipulas talks.

U.S. military forces have been training with the Guatemalans and have been involved in road building and health projects in conflict areas.

The pressure continues to build.

Appendix B

"The Cry for Land"

In February 1988, the Guatemalan Bishops Conference issued a joint pastoral letter on land reform called "The Cry for Land." The text of that letter follows. Translation is by Sally Hanlon. Several references to internal church documents have been deleted.

The cry for land is undoubtedly the strongest, most dramatic and most desperate cry heard in Guatemala. It bursts forth from millions of Guatemalan hearts yearning not only to possess the land, but to be possessed by it. It is a cry from the "People of Corn" who, on the one hand identify with furrows, sowing and harvest, and who on the other hand find themselves expelled from the land by an unjust and punitive system. They are like strangers in the land which belonged to them for thousands of years; they are considered second-class citizens in the nation forged by their extraordinary ancestors.

Perhaps there is no subject which awakens more fierce passion and gives rise to more radical and irreconcilable positions than does the subject of land ownership. But it is a subject which must be dealt with in an attempt to begin to solve the great problems troubling us.

Through this Pastoral Letter, we wish to invite all Guatemalans, especially those who profess to be Catholics, to reflect sincerely and in depth on this most difficult problem, letting ourselves be enlightened by the Word of God and establishing solid foundations on which we can build a better homeland.

Our letter is made up of three large sections: the agrarian problem in Guatemala, theological insights, and pastoral conclusions.

The Agrarian Problem in Guatemala

In fulfillment of our pastoral mission, we want to point out once again the critical situation of the majority of Guatemalans in rural areas. Like the Latin American Bishops at Puebla, we too feel and observe that "the most devastating and humiliating scourge" in Guatemala is the situation of dehumanizing poverty suffered by the *campesinos* [Guatemalan peasants] who painfully bring forth from Guatemalan soil a daily sustenance for themselves and their families. Rightfully called dehumanizing, this poverty is expressed by a high rate of illiteracy, by the mortality rate, by the lack of housing adequate to the dignity of the family, by unemployment and underemployment, by malnutrition and by other ills which we have carried with us for years.

The pitiable conditions lead us to question a system that produces inequities between those who enjoy possession of the goods of the earth even unto excess, and those who possess nothing or almost nothing. This breach between classes continues to widen, even amidst a people who profess to be Christian.

This is not the first time that we Guatemalan Bishops have denounced this injustice and labeled it as contrary to the Salvific Plan of God, our Father. Nor is this the first time that we have declared this the great challenge of our time in history, and that this marginalization endured by so many human beings is an appeal to us as people and as Christians. In our pastoral letters, we have already pointed out in the light of the Gospel that such an abysmal situation is not an accidental stage but rather the product of a sinful situation which is preventing a viable solution to the problem.

We seriously want to invite faithful Christians and people of good will to reflect upon the critical nature of the poverty and misery endured by campesinos, because we are convinced that no situation is so painful and calls more urgently for resolution. There are many problems afflicting our brothers and sisters in the rural areas in their long calvary of suffering. However, their dispossession of the land should be considered the nucleus of the social problem in Guatemala.

It is a fact that the majority of arable land is in the hands of a privileged few, while the majority of campesinos own no plot of land on which to sow their crops.

This situation, far from pointing toward a solution, becomes day by day more harsh and painful. Certainly the critical problem of land ownership is at the very heart of the propagation of injustice.

To attempt to get to the bottom of the social problem and its roots, we must recognize that the present situation has its origins in the system of land ownership imposed in colonial times. This is preserved with many of its flaws, vices and structures of unequal and unjust distribution, even to our own times.

During the colonial period, the policy of land ownership was determined by a two-pronged principle. On the one hand, giving over of large land extensions to a group of colonizers favored by the Spanish crown with "encomiendas" and "royal possessions" and on the other hand by exploiting the unpaid Indian labor force for the sake of production, the people could cultivate land for themselves.

The period of Independence accentuated by its arbitrary laws the concentration of land in the hands of the privileged few.

The situation was aggravated by the liberal reform of 1871 which, in order to promote coffee production, discouraged communal lands and the distributing of vast extensions among a middle class, giving origin to a powerful class of agricultural exporters.

During what has been called the second revolutionary government (1950-1954), a careful agrarian reform process was begun which, although flawed, has been the only serious attempt to modify an unjust structure. We all know the reaction which this produced among its detractors and how it was abruptly ended.

No one can deny the excessive inequality present today in regard to land ownership. The agrarian problem in Guatemala at the present time can be measured by merely considering the large landed estates and the small farms on the margin of which the great majority of campesinos who own no plot of land are situated.

Statistics drawn from the 1979 Agricultural Census demonstrate a dangerous concentration of land in a few hands with the majority of the population devoted to agriculture who are without adequate portions of land for tilling. The number of small landholders who own one block or less grew from 85,053 in 1964 to 247,090 in 1979. On the other hand, ever more land is concentrated in ever fewer hands, since the number of large landholders owning 855,800 acres (200 "caballerias") or more decreased from nine to four between 1964 and 1979.

According to data from the Third National Agricultural Census of 1979, the distribution by number and area of farms in Guatemala is as presented in the following chart:

Number and Size of Farms in Guatemala - 1979

Type of Farm	Number	Percent	Area[1]	Percent
Mini-farm[2]	240,132	37.81%	81,316	1.38%
Sub-family farm	301,736	47.51	890,229	15.15
Family farm	79,509	12.52	1,115,739	18.98
Medium multifamily	13,179	2.08	2,596,551	44.18
Large multifamily	478	0.08	1,193,611	20.31
Total	635,034	100.00%	5,877,446	100.00%

1. number of square blocks.
2. under 625 square yards.

This chart shows that 38% of the mini-farms constitute but 1.38% of the total land area in farms.

The situation is even more striking if it is taken into account that 85.32% of the farms (mini-farms and sub-family farms) constitute but 16.53% of the land area, while 2.16% of the farms (multifamily farms and large farms) constitute 64.51% of the area.

Such unequal land distribution results inevitably in grave socio-economic consequences and, above all, in a situation of violence among Guatemalan farmers.

The agricultural export sector, owning huge and fertile land areas, holds the best arable lands and the means of agricultural production. This elite in Guatemala produces and sells the goods which then receive the highest prices in the international market. These include coffee, cardamom, cotton, bananas, cattle and other traditional exports. This sector's economic solvency permits it to mechanize its cultivation process and to obtain bank credits with great facility. It must be recognized that it is the agricultural export sector which contributes most to obtaining the foreign exchange so urgently needed by Guatemala and which creates large numbers of jobs.

In contrast, there are very few campesino landowners, since the majority own no land. Those who do are devoted to subsistence farming on mini-plots where they sow only corn and beans. Large numbers find themselves obliged to rent land and are the victims of unfair speculation or are compelled to go down to the coast in unacceptable conditions. The difficulty of obtaining bank credits and the lack of adequate technical preparation leads them to exploit the land according to archaic systems, some of which are very damaging to the ecology. The majority do not benefit from any insurance system, nor do they have any possibilities of saving, so that a drought or a bad winter brings them to the brink of starvation and death.

It is no secret that the Guatemalan campesino is caught in a situation of desperate marginalization. The goods and services which the State is obliged to provide to *all* Guatemalans never reach the majority; neither do elementary school nor informal education; neither sanitary assistance nor any social security; nor any housing that has a modicum of hygiene and dignity.

Campesinos have extreme difficulty in trying to move beyond their marginalization because of scant opportunities, lack of preparation, and due to the very structure of Guatemalan society, which is organized for the benefit of a minority and with no regard for the vast majority of Guatemalans. It has come to seem natural for us to see the campesino or Indian dressed in rags, sick, dirty and despised. We call the damp, unliveable and unsanitary shacks "folklore" and tourist attractions. We are not shocked to see tiny children trudging off with their machete or hoe early in the morning beside the men, to carry out a hard and poorly paid day's work. We fail to react before the shameful spectacle of thousands of Indian peasants transported to the coastal plantations in trucks without security nor even minimal comfort. This attitude on the part of those of us who are not campesinos toward our Guatemalan brothers and sisters is but a reflection of our Nation's social and economic structure. The constitutional precept which establishes the equality of all citizens is not honored. Public funds are principally aimed for the benefit of those of us who use the highways, airports, electric lights, universities and hospitals. There are several million Guatemalans who don't benefit from these services, although they have contributed their share of taxes, have been obliged to do military service and to lose millions of hours of work-hours in the Civil Defense Patrols. A huge social debt weighs upon the entire Nation.

In our society the campesino is frequently exploited in a ruthless and inhumane way. The campesino continues to be the cheapest and most cruelly exploited labor force. It is obvious that the legal minimum wage of Q4.50 [daily minimum of $1.50] is insufficient nowadays, given the high cost of living. And although there are some employers who pay more than the minimum legal wage and organize a system of loans and benefits, many still resist paying even the minimum wage. Then there are those who find a way to get around it, taking advantage of the extreme need in which the campesinos find themselves. To argue these cases for the law of supply and demand is, from every point of view, unjust and inhumane. Human work is not a marketable item!

Some people's attitudes toward campesinos are so harsh that in order to increase their profits, they go as far as eradicating the *mozo colono* tradition (one's right to work a given piece of land on a plantation or farm because one's family has served the plantation/farm for generations). This pre-capitalist, anachronistic and paternalistic relationship provides the campesino, who has lived for generations on a particular plantation, a certain statute guaranteeing him a kind of stability and right to work on that property and to continue cultivating certain strips of land for his own use. Certainly this represents a burden to the employer or owner, because it carries with it some minimal social responsibilities and honors certain rights. Even this, miserable and imperfect as it is, they seek to wipe out. Many landowners exert pressures and resort to clever tricks, not excluding armed violence, to discourage the *mozos colonos* and to force these campesinos to leave the farm in which they and their parents and grandparents were born and where they have established their home. It just so happens that it is easier and less complicated to bring in work crews each year at harvest time in a system which adds to the impoverishment of campesinos.

Over the course of many decades, a grave problem has been generated in Guatemala by those who work as intermediaries and/or negotiators of legal-administrative matters before government institutions, as by middlemen in agricultural commerce, those who hire or bring in laborers. These, too, participate in the exploitation of campesinos and in their impoverishment. It can be said that this is an institutionalized problem, since it is commonly accepted by the society. It is sad to see that even liberal professionals, unscrupulous businessmen and landowners participate in these schemes which deepen the wounds of their own people.

We should not be surprised that this unjust social situation is one of the reasons why campesinos flee from their places of origin and migrate to the city, seeing it as a refuge from their misery and as a possible solution to their extreme poverty. The campesino thus arrives in town or city, swelling the ranks of the unemployed, multiplying the slum areas, and many times falling into the webs and vice of delinquency. It is not unusual that campesinos also lose the only possession they have left, their Catholic faith. In this way millions of campesino families have been violently forced to flee their lands to seek refuge beyond their own homeland.

The grave problems which municipalities face in providing indispensable public services will continue to increase daily as campesinos abandon their *trabajaderos* [workplaces]. Simultaneously hospital health service, educational service in government schools, and all public services generally will become more inadequate and insufficient.

Violence in the rural area is common. The very situation of desperation is a source of many tensions that are a shout of protest and a cry of desperation from hundreds of thousands of people. Nothing is solved if we merely try to place blame on agitators or leaders, since the root of the evil is in the social situation itself. All of us inhabitants of our country must open our eyes to the gravity of the problem.

We observe joyfully that the campesinos are daily reaching a greater awareness of their rights and of their own dignity. This is an irreversible move forward and, despite the continuing and brutal repression to which they have been subjected, theirs is a legitimate cry and action in defense of the land.

But we fear that without proper accommodation for these hopes and if mechanisms are not established for responding quickly and effectively to their request, an outburst of violence may result with unforeseen consequences. We have in mind the painful case of Panzos in Alta Verapaz. It is a tragedy and a crime which we still remember and condemn, since we know well that just ten years ago more than a hundred Kekchi Indians were massacred over land problems. This could happen again in any place and at any moment. The multitudinous demonstrations held in many parts of Guatemala are an indication of the troublesome situation in the rural area. Because of it, we repeat again with Pope John Paul II: "To forestall any extremism and to consolidate an authentic peace, there is no better way than to return their dignity to those who suffer injustice, contempt and misery" (John Paul II, Homily at Campo de Marte, March 7, 1983).

In the light of God's Word and the Church Magisterium, we want to offer to the faithful and to all people of good will a word of guidance regarding the Christian meaning of land ownership.

Theological Insights

In the Bible the subject of land is important, because from the dawn of creation to the Apocalypse the human person develops in a particular land, God's gift and the habitation of God with people.

Scripture describes for us the origin of humanity, saying that it was created in the image of God (Gen. 1:26). This is the theological basis for human dignity. God also blessed that humanity created as man and woman (Gen. 1:27) that it might multiply, filling and submitting the earth. The fruits of the earth were given them as food (Gen. 1:27). The earth is, then, according to God's plan, humanity's world.

Man and woman belong to the earth (Gen. 2:7) and it belongs to them because right after creating them God charges them with tilling and caring for the earth (Gen. 2:15). Thus farmwork appears as the essential task defining and situating the human person in the world and before God.

Many Scripture texts express humanity's joy at the fruit of their labors on the earth and their gratitude to God for the divine blessing. When the earth gives its harvest, men and women know that God is blessing them (Ps. 67:7, 85:13).

The joy with which people gather up the first fruits and conclude the harvest was in the ancient people of God an occasion for the family to make a pilgrimage to the sanctuary of the Lord and to celebrate there a fiesta in God's honor (Deut. 16:1–15).

These agricultural feasts, continued now in the completely new light of our Christian Easter and Pentecost feasts, teach us to rejoice before the Lord for the goods of the earth, and show us that we should share with those who have less of the abundance with which God has blessed us.

The Lord promises his oppressed people in Egypt that God will guide them to a good and spacious land yielding milk and honey (Ex. 3:8). Thus the promise made to Abraham is gathered up again (Gen. 12:1).

When the Israelites offered the first fruits of the earth, he remembered that the earth and those fruits were a gift from God (Deut. 26: 9-10). When the people came into possession of the earth, each tribe was assigned its territory according to its inhabitants: "You shall increase the legacy of the numerous and reduce that of the meager" (Numbers 26:54). In this way no individual nor tribe will come into possession of the land by depriving others of their livelihood.

The earth does not belong to men but to the Lord, and what each one calls his property is in reality the portion to which he is entitled in order to make a living. The earth is the Lord's and the bounty thereof, the world and those who inhabit therein (Ps. 24:1).

The voice of the prophets was raised to denounce those who hoarded the earth with greed to the detriment of the poor and destitute: "Woe unto you who gather house upon house and field upon field, annexing until you occupy the whole place and are the sole inhabitants of the country! Thus has the Lord of hosts sworn to my ears: 'Many great and beautiful homes shall be left abandoned, without inhabitants' " (Is. 5:8-9). "Woe unto those who meditate upon evil. They covet fields and steal them, homes and usurp them; they do violence to a man and to his house, to an individual and his inheritance. Behold I am preparing an hour of misfortune against you who do this from which you shall never escape" (Mi. 2:1-2).

The prophet's voice was also raised against those who did not pay or who gave unjust wages to their workers. "Woe unto the one who builds his house without justice and his foundations without righteousness! He takes advantage of his neighbor and does not pay the neighbor for his work" (Jer. 22:13). "These are those who, resting upon marble beds, lounging upon their couches, drink wine from large cups, anoint themselves with the best of perfumes, but care nothing for the ruin of my people" (Amos 6:4-6).

This denunciation of avarice and of the excessive wealth attained by the hoarding of land and by the paying of unjust wages is also repeated in the New Testament writings. "You rich, weep and cry out over the disgraces which are about to fall upon you! Look, the salary you have not paid to the workers who harvested your fields is shouting; and the cries of the harvesters have reached the ears of the Lord of hosts. You have lived in luxury upon the earth and given yourselves over to pleasures" (James 5:1,4-5).

Jesus, the Son of God, Lord of heaven and earth, had nowhere to lay his head (Luke 9:58). He being rich, became poor for our sake. This poverty freed him to carry out his mission: "To evangelize the poor" (Luke 4:18).

Jesus does not present himself as a judge or arbiter in the distribution of legacies. On one occasion he rejects such a request in order to make evident that earthly goods do not guarantee one's existence.

Then he tells the parable of the man whose fields gave forth such an abundant harvest that he had to put up new, much larger grain bins in order to store it. He thought that with this he would have enough to live for many years, but that night he died (Luke 12:13-21). This is why Jesus also calls down woe upon the rich and upon those who are full (Luke 6:24-25). And he describes money as "unjust" (Luke 16:9) when there is at the origin of great wealth the exploitation of the weak. That is why Jesus commands the rich who want to follow him to place their wealth at the service of the needy: "Sell what you have and give alms" (Luke 12:33).

The concept of "alms," so frequent in the New Testament, should be correctly understood. It was an ancient practice by which the most powerful members of a population took charge of the neediest in the community—the orphans, widows, strangers—providing for them a means of subsistence. The concept, then, expresses the moral responsibility of one who has more toward those without possessions (Deut. 15:7-8, 10-11).

The New Testament affirms that the world was created by the One who is the Word of God and that without Him nothing of what exists was created (John 1:3). This Word of God became flesh, truly a human being in Jesus (John 1:14). In such a way Jesus can be called the "first-born of all creation." It is not that he was the first of creatures, but that all that exists finds its meaning in Him, "because in Him were created all things and everything was created by Him and for Him" (Col. 1:15-16).

Because of this, Christ's redeeming work affects not only the group of believers of humanity alone; but rather by his death and resurrection, Christ reconciled all things with God, "pacifying, by the blood of His cross, everything on earth and in the heavens" (Col. 1:20). Christ's Paschal

Mystery has transformed human beings from sinners to the just who live for God (Rom. 6:11). But creation has been redeemed, too, together with people, and groans in "the hope of being freed from its servitude to corruption in order to participate in the glorious freedom of the children of God" (Rom. 8:20-21). This liberation begins for creation when the goods of the earth cease to be instruments of human rivalry and exploitation in order to become a means of friendship and communion.

The effect of the transformation brought about by Christ's Paschal Mystery is palpable in the first Christian community called together by the Risen Lord in the power of the Spirit. It is true that in this community there is deceit and sin, as in the case of Ananias and Safira (Acts 5:1-11); however, the testimony of friendship prevails, a friendship which unites all the believers: "the multitude of believers had but one heart and a single soul. No one called their belongings their own, but rather everything was held in common among them. . . . There was in their midst no one in need, because all those who had fields or homes sold them, brought in the money from the sale and set it at the feet of the apostles, and they distributed it to each one according to their need" (Acts 4:32-35).

Faith in the Risen Lord and the friendship which thus results lead to a new earth in which justice is at home (II Peter 3:13). "At the time there will be a new heaven and a new earth where there shall be no death nor tears, nor cries nor fatigue, because the old world shall have passed away" (Apoc. 21:1-4).

That hope should encourage our awareness today so that in the meantime we may make of this earth a place of togetherness in justice and equity.

The biblical teaching concerning land ownership has been studied and reflected upon in depth since the Church began. The Holy Fathers have left us an impressive wealth of thought and examples of action on topics such as the meaning of property, the role of earthly goods and the demands of social justice.

The Church has always recognized the right of all people to own property sufficient for themselves and for their family. However, this right to property "constitutes for no one an unconditional and absolute right. There is no reason to reserve for one's own exclusive use what goes beyond our need while others are lacking essentials."

This is the teaching which, like a river of pure water, flows through the history of the Church and which, in the recent period of Vatican Council II and under recent Popes in their social encyclicals has been repeated tirelessly. "God has destined the earth and everything she contains for the use of all human beings and all people."

There is special vigor in the thought expressed by John Paul II during his inaugural address at the Third General Conference of Latin American bishops: "Upon all private property there is a *grave social responsibility* [literally, a social *mortgage*].

Because of this, the right to private property is not an absolute right, but rather a conditional one, limited by a broader and more universal principle: God has created all things for the use and benefit of all human beings, with no distinction whatsoever.

The Holy Fathers have also referred directly to land distribution. Thus, for example, St. Ambrose declares: "It is not part of your [own] goods that you give to the poor, but rather what belongs to them. Because you have appropriated to yourself what was given for the use of everyone. The earth has been given for the whole world and not merely for the wealthy." St. John Chrisostum is even more explicit: "God never made some rich and others poor. God gave the earth to everyone. The whole earth belongs to the Lord, and the fruits of the earth should be available [literally 'common'] to all." The *mine* and *thine* are motive and cause for discord. Community of goods is therefore a form of existence more adequate to our nature than is private property itself.

During his apostolic trips to Latin America, Pope John Paul II has been able to see and touch our reality; and since having this direct experience, he has strengthened Church doctrine on the subject of land.

When he experienced personally that a timid application of doctrinal principles resulted in conflictive social situations in which a large number of people had no access to the goods necessary for their human fulfillment, he expressed to the campesinos in Cuilapan, Mexico, the need for profound reforms: "As for you who are responsible for [whole] peoples, you powerful classes who sometimes hold uncultivated the land that hides the daily bread needed by so many: the human conscience, the conscience of nations, the cry of the destitute, and above all the Voice of God, the voice of the Church repeat with me: It is not just, nor is it human, nor Christian to continue on with certain situations which are clearly unjust."

In Recife, Brazil, John Paul II said to the farmers: "The earth is a gift from God, a gift God makes to every human being, men and women, whom God wants gathered together in a single family and related to one another with a spirit of friendship. It is not right, therefore, because it is not in harmony with God's plan, to use this gift in such a way that the earth's benefits favor just a few, leaving others, the immense majority, excluded" (homily at the Mass celebrated for farmers).

Today Guatemalan campesinos have an ever-clearer awareness that they live in what Leo XIII and Paul VI called *undeserved misery*. Because of this, they are raising their voices from all over the country, urging those responsible for the nation to "put into effect daring and profoundly innovative transformations . . . to bring about, without further delay, urgent reforms" (John Paul II to the campesinos in Cuilapan) so that the goods created by God may reach everyone with equity, according to the rule of justice, inseparable from charity.

Pastoral Conclusions

Throughout these reflections we have reviewed the injustices the unequal land ownership in Guatemala engenders. We also have tried to sketch in the light of scriptural reflection and Church teaching, the divine plan for God's children. As shepherds of the Church in Guatemala, we have the grave obligation given us by our ministry, to denounce the situation which is at the root of our dehumanizing poverty. We Christians should not only concern ourselves with the problems of our nation, but above all "involve ourselves" in them. The first step will be to become aware of the situation suffered by our campesino brothers and sisters.

As we pointed out in 1984: "An evil distribution of property, immense extensions of uncultivated or insufficiently cultivated land make of our people a hungry, sickly people with a high mortality rate" (message of the Guatemalan Espiscopate, May 9, 1984).

In Pope John Paul II's encyclical "Laboren Exercens," we read a description/denunciation which finds in Guatemala a desperate case in point: "In some developing countries, millions of people find themselves obliged to cultivate others' land and are exploited by large landowners, with no hope of managing to own some day even a tiny plot of land of their own. Long working days of heavy physical labor are paid miserably. Cultivated lands are abandoned by their owners, legal titles for possession of a small plot, cultivated over many years, are not taken into account or are without defense in the face of the 'hunger for land' of more powerful individuals and groups."

All these situations naturally provoke the outcry of the campesinos for their rights; but we know (because we have such recent experience that we cannot forget it) that the campesino's cry has been stifled by the power of arms. Thousands of campesinos have been killed in Guatemala merely for having attempted a change of structure. Since then, as a result of this terrible repression suffered by Guatemalans, campesino organizations of whatever type are viewed with suspicion and there are no lack of coercive measures to suppress them. At this level there should be mentioned the role — forced [compliance] in practice — of the Civil Defense Patrols which enormously limit the campesinos' right of association. It is not unusual to learn that campesinos have been hunted down or "disappeared." This list has become by now one of the most shameful and tragic in our history.

Unfortunately, as we pointed out above, there is a painful lack of legislation when it comes to defending the campesino and his rights or to really promoting them effectively. On the contrary, Guatemalan legislation seems designed to maintain a system of land ownership which benefits the large landowner and those who control economic and military power to the detriment of the campesinos and Indians. This legislation forms the basis and the legal framework for the unjust situation experienced in Guatemala, as we already stated several years ago in our Pastoral Letter, "United in Hope."

Episcopal Guidelines

This entire list of negative circumstances cannot cause us as Christians to remain passive out of disappointment or discouragement. Our response must be a positive one. Evil and all its consequences have been overcome by Christ, who triumphed over sin and death. It is up to us to take this redemption to the sinful structures of our national situation.

But this is a task that can only be carried out effectively if all of us do our part generously. Because of this, the first requirement is SOLIDARITY. Only insofar as we feel ourselves brothers and sisters in solidarity with one another can such a critical problem as the ownership and exploitation of land in Guatemala find channels for solution. Solidarity is the opposite of egotistical individualism, since it makes us think of others at the same time as we think of our own needs. It makes us seek a solution to the problems of our neighbors. It has its basis in the Christian meaning of friendship, since solidarity is based precisely on a fundamental truth of Christianity: we are all brothers and sisters because we are children of the same God, we are gifted with the same dignity, we enjoy the same rights and we are called to the same glorification with God.

At times of crisis, such as the one we are living in in Guatemala, there is a tendency to forget everyone else and just try to save ourselves (*salvese quien pueda*) which kills all sense of solidarity and throws people into a frenetic search for egotistical satisfactions leading to extremes of consumerism. We must react against such an orientation in our life and action, appealing to the great principles of faith.

Another important aspect in the search for genuine and adequate solutions to the grave problems of land ownership is the effort to reach a high degree of development. But this will be not merely an economic development. Rather, it should be an authentic integral human and social development as expressed by Pope Paul VI in his Encyclical "The Progress of Peoples."

We should struggle so that this development may reach everyone, not just a privileged group. Development should reach the entire people.

If any sector should be privileged, let it be the campesino or Indian people, not simply because it is the majority of the Guatemalan population, but also because of a basic sense of justice, in order to compensate in some way for the centuries of abandonment they have endured, as if they were citizens of a second or inferior class. Guatemala will not progress as it should as long as, with inconceivable myopia, it tries to keep marginalized the campesino and worker sectors, "the dynamizing force in the building up of a more participative society."

In effect, this has been one of the causes of Guatemala's greatest tragedy; preventing, out of egotism and irrational fear, the full use of the campesino potential to make the land produce abundantly.

If this sleeping giant is not invited and prepared to participate in the building up of a better Guatemala, it will awaken embittered by the contempt heaped upon it over many centuries and may become a source of even more painful and violent conflict.

Nothing we have spoken of can come about unless we accept the idea that a change of sinful and obsolete social structures is necessary and urgent in Guatemala. We want to make our own the strong words of John Paul II in his historic message at Oaxaca, Mexico, in 1979: "Real, efficacious measures must be put in practice at the local, national and international levels along the broad lines set out in the encyclical MATER ET MAGISTRA."

The Pope invites us to follow the broad guidelines set out by John XXIII's encyclical MATER ET MAGISTRA which has been called the campesino's "Magna Carta." This encyclical, in effect, highlights the emphasis that should be given to the agricultural sector when it says: "Now in order to attain a proportionate development among the different sectors of the economy, it is also absolutely essential [that there be] an economic policy in regard to farming, followed by public, political and economic authorities, who must deal with the following ideas: fiscal responsibility [taxation], credits, social security, prices, publicity and complementary industries and, finally, the perfecting of the farming enterprise structure."

In harmony with church doctrine and with the needs of Guatemala, the following measures, urgently needed to improve the situation, may be highlighted:

1. To legislate in view of an equitable land distribution, beginning with the vast government properties and "properties insufficiently cultivated, in favor of those able to make them fruitful" (G.S. 71)
2. To facilitate the presenting of additional titles for lands which the campesinos have been cultivating for years

3. To guarantee legally the defense of campesinos and refugees so that they will not be stripped of their lands

4. To defend the campesinos against speculation in the renting of lands to be cultivated

5. To assure that campesinos receive a just and equitable price, protecting them from voracious and unscrupulous middlemen

6. To give an adequate farming education to the greatest possible number of campesinos, so that they may improve their methods of cultivating and may be able to diversify their crops

7. To grant the greatest possible facilities for bank credits and for acquiring seeds, fertilizers, and other materials and farming tools needed

8. To increase the salary of the campesinos in accord with human dignity and their family responsibilities

9. To open up channels and to create mechanisms so that the campesino can participate actively and directly in the local, regional, national and even international marketplace

10. To diminish the indirect taxes on the purchasing of products for farmwork

11. To create direct taxes for large land extensions proportionate to the size of the lands

12. To organize some kind of protective measures for campesinos against poor harvests and work accidents

13. To stimulate and protect campesino organizations in defense of their rights and to increase their farm production.

We cannot resort to violence because it is neither evangelical nor Christian, but rather generates further violence in an endless spiral. As Christians, we have more confidence in the power of those who are non-violent than in the brute force of those who place all their trust in armed homicides.

A second characteristic is that the change of structures should be brought about legally. We advocate an adequate legislation which takes as its goal the common welfare and defense of the campesino who, as we have pointed out repeatedly, is in practice the weakest, poorest and most defenseless sector in our society. We are convinced that measures which are in fact outside the law aggravate the problem (like invading land—far from solving the agrarian problem, it increases it) and lead to explosions which are impossible to control.

We Christians are peaceful and builders of peace. We trust in the foundation of the law, in the value of what is reasonable, and above all, in the transforming power of love. And based upon this conviction, we demand that the changes which are indispensable for seeking adequate solutions to such an enormous problem, be carried out urgently though without the haste which might diminish the reasonableness, efficacy and credibility of the measures. We are aware that something which has been structured over the course of many centuries cannot be changed overnight. However, it is essential to delay no longer than necessary, as delay might aggravate the agrarian problem even further.

Conclusions

We have tried to promote a reflection which is deep, serene, sincere and constructive on one of the most serious and complex problems in our Guatemalan panorama. In our judgment, this is the fundamental problem in the social structure in Guatemala. To solve it will mean having achieved, through a difficult but patriotic process, a basic change in Guatemalan history.

We have thus shed light on this reality with the Word of God and the teaching of the Church, demonstrating that it is not something foreign to our pastoral mission, but rather something that falls within the lines of our work as shepherds of the Church. Neither the sufferings nor the errors of the people entrusted to us can be beyond our concern.

For all these reasons, we have the hope that our faithful will read this Pastoral Letter attentively and will study it, trying to discover the very positive perspective that it offers for the future of our Guatemala. We also have the hope that everyone will commit themselves with a fraternal spirit to carrying out the tremendous task implied in finding an adequate and peaceful solution to such a grave problem.

Our pastoral invitation is sent with great hope to the Government, to political parties, to Guatemala's productive forces, to the means of social communication and to the private sector; also to Catholic lay movements and to the Indians and campesinos, inviting them to join forces fraternally and peacefully in an effort which calls for the commitment of every Guatemalan.

We recognize that in the final analysis the most difficult thing is personal conversion. Conversion means a "turning around," a radical change. As long as one's only goal is profit, to grow rich, ambition for money or power, it is impossible to understand these truths which we have desired to bring to mind, and to see with Christian eyes the reality which must be transformed.

We have presented the human and moral aspects of the problem rather than delving more deeply into the technical and practical aspects which go beyond our mission. Our pastoral service is limited to a posing of the problem in the light of human dignity, the common good and Christian love.

In concluding this Letter, we ask God, through the intercessions of the Virgin Mary, Mother of all people, who moves our hearts and illumines our understanding, that setting aside every violent, revengeful and biased attitude, we may give a worthy, courageous and Christian response to the tremendous "CRY FOR LAND."

Guatemala de la Asuncion
February 29, 1988

Prospero Penados del Barrio
Archbishop of Guatemala

Rodolfo Quezada Toruno
President of the Guatemalan Episcopal Conference

And the Bishops of Guatemala

Appendix C

Peace Accords

Caraballeda Declaration

In 1983, four nations began meeting in an attempt to find a peaceful solution to the problems of Central America. The four became known as the Contadora Group—Mexico, Venezuela, Colombia, and Panama. In 1985, they were joined by the Contadora Support Group—Argentina, Brazil, Peru, and Uruguay.

The Caraballeda Declaration was issued by the eight Contadora nations in January 1986. It was subsequently endorsed by the presidents of all five Central American countries.

Any permanent solution to the Central American conflict must be based on fair and balanced principles, which express traditional values and the desire of the Latin American peoples for civilized coexistence. It is for this reason that the Ministers of the Contadora Group and of the Group of Support have determined the following principles for peace in Central America:

1. A Latin American solution: meaning that the solution to Latin American problems must come from, and receive the support of, the region itself, so that it will not be included in the East-West strategic conflict.
2. Self-determination: meaning the independence of each of the Latin American countries to determine its own form of social and political organization, establishing at a domestic level the type of government which is freely chosen by the entire population.

3. Non-intervention in the affairs of other states: which means that no country will be able to influence, directly or by acting indirectly through a third party, the political situation of the Latin American states, or in any way that affects their sovereignty.
4. Territorial integrity: meaning the recognition of limits of action for each of the countries, within which each country can exercise its sovereignty and outside which each country must observe a strict compliance with the norms of international law.
5. Pluralistic democracy: meaning the right to universal suffrage by free and regular elections, supervised by independent national organizations: a multiparty system that will allow the legal and organized representation of all kinds of political action and thought. A government of the majority, ensuring the basic liberties and rights of all citizens and the respect of political minorities according to the society's constitutional order.
6. No presence of arms or military bases which threaten peace and security in the region.
7. No undertaking of military actions by countries in the region or with ties to the region, which may present a threat to the region or its peace.
8. No presence of foreign troops or advisers.
9. No political, logistical, or military support to any group intending to subvert or destabilize the constitutional order of any Latin American state through force or terrorist acts of any kind.
10. Observance of human rights: meaning the unrestricted defense of civil, political and religious liberties, thus ensuring the complete material and spiritual fulfillment of all citizens.

Guatemala Accords

In August 1987, the presidents of all five Central American countries signed the Guatemala Accords, indicating their intent to implement steps which would provide peace, stability, and democracy.

The Governments of the Republic of Costa Rica, Guatemala, Honduras and Nicaragua, determined to achieve the objectives and to develop the principles established in the United Nations Charter and the Charter of the Organization of the American States, the Document of Objectives, the Caraballeda Message for Peace, Security and Democracy in Central America, the Guatemala Declaration, the Punta del Este Communique, the Declaration of Panama, the Esquipulas Declaration, and the Contadora Treaty Proposal for Peace and Cooperation in Central America of July 6, 1986, have agreed on the following procedure for establishing a firm and lasting peace in Central America:

National Reconciliation

Dialogue. To urgently carry out, in those cases where deep divisions have resulted within society, steps for national reconciliation which would allow for popular participation with full guarantees in authentic political processes of a democratic nature based on justice, freedom and democracy. Towards this end, to create those mechanisms which, in accordance with the law, would allow for dialogue with opposition groups. For this purpose, the corresponding Governments will initiate a dialogue-with all unarmed internal political opposition groups and with those who have availed themselves of amnesty.

Amnesty. In each Central American country, except where the International Commission of Verification and Follow-up determines that such a measure is not necessary, an Amnesty decree will be issued containing all the provisions for the guarantee of the inviolability of life; as well as freedom in all its forms, property and the security of the persons to whom these decrees apply. Simultaneous with the issuing of the amnesty decree by the Government, the irregular forces of the respective country will place in freedom all persons in their power.

National Reconciliation Commission. In order to verify the compliance with the commitments that the five Central American Governments subscribed to by the signing of this document, concerning amnesty, cease-fire, democratization and free elections, a National Reconciliation Commission will be established whose duties will be to verify the actual carrying out in practice of the national reconciliation process, as well as the full exercise of all civil and political rights of Central American citizens guaranteed in this document. The National Reconciliation Commission will be comprised of a delegate and an alternate delegate from the executive branch; a bishop delegate recommended by the Episcopal Conference, and chosen by the Government from a list of three candidates which should be presented [by the conference] within a period of fifteen days upon receival of a formal invitation. This invitation will be made by the Governments within five working days from the signing of this document.

The same procedure will be used to select a delegate and alternate delegate from the legally registered political opposition parties. The said list of three [candidates] should be presented within the same above-mentioned period.

In addition, each Central American Government will chose an outstanding citizen, outside of public office and not pertaining to the party in power, and his respective alternate, to be part of this commission.

The decree, which puts into effect the agreements for the nomination of the members of the respective national commissions, shall be communicated immediately to the other Central American Governments.

Exhortation for the Cessation of Hostilities. The Governments make a vehement appeal so that in the States of the area currently suffering from the activity of irregular or insurgent groups, a cessation of hostilities be arranged. The Governments of these States commit themselves to undertake all the necessary steps for achieving an effective cease-fire within the constitutional framework.

Negotiations on Matters Relating to Security, Verification, Control and Limitation of Armaments. The Governments of the five Central American states, with the participation of the Contadora group in exercise of its role as mediator, will continue negotiations on the points still pending in the Contadora Treaty Proposal for Peace and Cooperation in Central America concerning security, verification and control.

In addition, these negotiations will entail measures for the disarmament of the irregular forces who are willing to accept the amnesty decrees.

Refugees and Displaced Persons. The Governments of Central America commit themselves to give urgent attention to the groups of refugees and displaced persons brought about by the regional crisis, through protection and assistance, particularly in areas of education, health, work and security, and whenever voluntary and individually expressed, to facilitate in the repatriation, resettlement and relocation [of these persons]. They also commit themselves to request assistance for Central American refugees and displaced persons from the international community, both directly through bilateral or multilateral agreements, as well as through the United Nations High Commissioner for Refugees and other organizations and agencies.

Cooperation, Democracy and Freedom for Peace and Development. In the climate of freedom guaranteed by democracy, the Central American countries will adopt the intensification of development in order to achieve more egalitarian and poverty-free societies. Consolidation of democracy presupposes the creation of a system of economic and social justice and well-being. To achieve these objectives the Governments will jointly seek special economic support from the international community.

Free Elections. Once the conditions inherent to every democracy are established, free, pluralist and honest elections shall be held as a joint expression of the Central American states to seek reconciliation and lasting peace for its peoples. Elections will be held for a Central American parliament, whose founding was proposed in the Esquipulas Declaration of May 25, 1986. In pursuit of the above-mentioned objectives, the leaders expressed their will to progress in the formation of this parliament and agreed that the Preparatory Commission of the Central American Parliament shall conclude its deliberations and submit to the Central American Presidents the respective treaty proposal within 150 days.

These elections will take place simultaneously in all the countries throughout Central America in the first half of 1988, on a date mutually agreed to by the Presidents of the Central American states. These elections will be subject to vigilance by the appropriate electoral bodies. The respective governments commit themselves to extend an invitation to the Organization of American States and to the United Nations, as well as to governments of third states, to send observers who shall bear witness that the electoral processes have been held in accordance with the strictest norms of equality, of access of all political parties to the media, as well as full guarantees for public demonstrations and other kinds of proselytizing propaganda.

The appropriate founding treaty shall be submitted for approval or ratification in the five countries so that the elections for the Central American parliament can be held within the period indicated in this paragraph. After the elections for the Central American parliament have been held, equally free and democratic elections shall be held with international observers and the same guarantees in each country, to name popular representatives to municipalities, congresses and legislative assemblies and the presidencies of the republics. These elections will be held according to the proposed calendars and within the periods established in the current political Constitutions.

Cessation of Assistance to Irregular Forces or Insurrectionist Movements. The Governments of the five Central American states shall request the Governments of the region, and the extra-regional governments which openly or covertly provide military, logistical, financial, propagandistic aid in manpower, armaments, munitions and equipment to irregular forces or insurrectionist movements to cease this aid, as an indispensable element for achieving a stable and lasting peace in the region.

The above does not include assistance for repatriation, or in lieu thereof, the reassigning of the assistance necessary for those persons having belonged to these groups or forces to become reintegrated into normal life. Likewise, the irregular forces or insurgent groups who operate in Central America will be asked to abstain, in yearnings for a true Latin American spirit, from receiving such assistance.

These petitions will be made in accordance with the provisions of the Document of Objectives regarding the elimination of arms traffic, whether it be inter-regional or extra-regional, intended for persons, organizations or groups attempting to destabilize the governments of the Central American countries.

The Non-Use of Territory to Invade Other States. The five countries which signed this document reaffirm their commitment to prevent the use of their own territory and to neither render or permit military or logistical support to persons, organizations, or groups attempting to destabilize the governments of the Central American countries.

Democratization. The Governments commit themselves to promote an authentic democratic, pluralist and participatory process that includes the promotion of social justice; respect for human rights, [state] sovereignty, the territorial integrity of states and the right of all nations to freely determine, without outside interference of any kind, its economic, political, and social model; and to carry out in a verifiable manner those measures leading to the establishment, or in their instances, the improvement of representative and pluralist democratic systems which would provide guarantees for the organization of political parties, effective popular participation in the decision making process, and to ensure free access to different currents of opinion, to honest electoral processes and newspapers based on the full exercise of citizens' rights.

For the purpose of verifying the good faith in the development of this democratization process, it will be understood that there shall exist complete freedom of press, television, and radio. This complete freedom will include the opening and maintaining in operations of communications media for all ideological groups, and the operation of this media without prior censorship.

Complete political pluralism should be manifest. In this regard, political groupings shall have broad access to communications media, full exercise of the right of association and the right to manifest publicly the exercise of their right to free speech, be it oral, written or televised, as well as freedom of movement by members of political parties in order to proselytize.

Likewise, those Governments of Central America, which have in effect a state of exception, siege, or emergency [law] shall terminate that state and reestablish the full exercise of all constitutional guarantees.

International Verification and Follow-up

International Verification and Follow-up Commission. An international verification and follow-up commission will be established comprised of the Secretary Generals of the Organization of American States and theUnited Nations or their representatives, as well as the Foreign Ministers of Central America, of the Contadorá Group and the Support Group. This commission will have the duties of verifying and following up the compliance with the commitments undertaken in this document, as well as the support and facilities given to the mechanisms for reconciliation and verification and follow-up. In order to strengthen the efforts of the International Commission of Verification and Follow-up, the Governments of the five Central American states shall issue declarations of support for [the commission's] work. All nations interested in promoting the cause of freedom, democracy, and peace in Central America can adhere to these declarations.

The five Governments shall offer all the necessary facilities for full compliance with the duties of verification and follow-up of the National Reconciliation Commission of each country and of the International Commission of Verification and Follow-up.

Calendar for the Implementation of Agreements. Within a period of fifteen days from the signing of this document, the Foreign Ministers of Central America will meet as the Executive Committee to regulate, promote and make feasible compliance with the agreements contained herein, and to organize the working commissions so that, henceforth, the processes leading to compliance with the contracted commitments may be initiated within the stipulated periods by means of consultations, undertakings and other mechanisms deemed necessary. Ninety days from the signing of this document, the commitments pertaining to Amnesty, Cease-Fire, Democratization, Cessation of Assistance to Irregular Forces or Insurrectionist Movements, and the Non-Use of Territory to Invade Other States, will enter into force simultaneously and publicly as defined herein.

One hundred twenty days from the signing of this document, the International Commission for Verification and Follow-up will analyze the progress [made] in the compliance with the agreements provided for herein.

After 150 days, the five Central American presidents will meet and receive a report from the International Commission of Verification and Follow-up and they will make the pertinent decisions.

Final Provisions. The points included in this document form part of a harmonious and indivisible whole. The signing of [the document] incursan obligation, accepted in good faith, to simultaneously comply with the agreement in the established periods.

We, the Presidents of the five States of Central America, with the political will to respond to the longings for peace of our peoples, sign [this document] in the City of Guatemala, on the seventh day of August of 1987.

> Oscar Arias Sanchez
> Jose Napoleon Duarte
> Vinicio Cerezo Arevalo
> Jose Azcona Hoyo
> Daniel Ortega Saavedra

Appendix D

MAP OF GUATEMALA

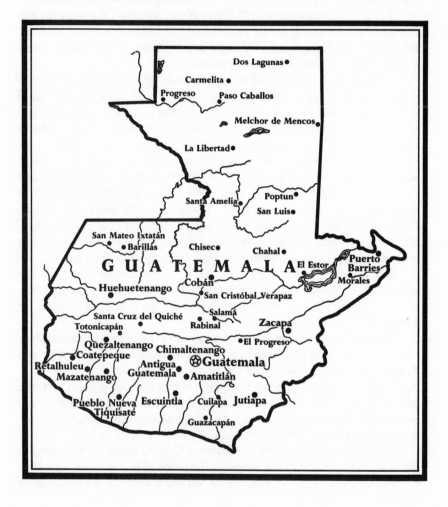

Appendix E

MAP OF CENTRAL AMERICA

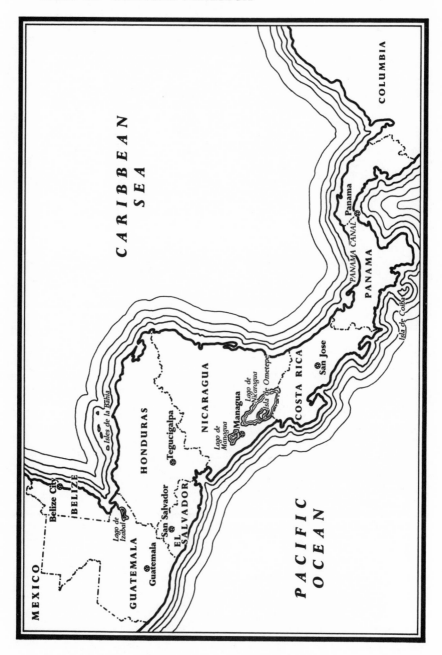

Bibliography

Barney, Gerald O. *Global 2000: The Report to the President.* Washington, D.C.: Seven Locks Press, 1980.

Berryman, Phillip. *Liberation Theology: The Essential Facts about the Revolutionary Movement in Latin America and Beyond.* New York: Pantheon Books, 1987.

Berryman, Phillip. *The Religious Roots of Rebellion: Christians in Central America.* Maryknoll, N.Y.: Orbis Books, 1984.

Blachman, Morris J., William M. LeoGrande, and Kenneth E. Sharpe, editors. *Confronting Revolution: Security through Diplomacy in Central America.* New York: Pantheon Books,1986.

Black, Eric. *Rethinking the Cold War.* Minneapolis: Paradigm Press, 1988.

Buckley, Tom. *Violent Neighbors: El Salvador, Central America, and the United States.* New York: Times Books, 1984.

Fagen, Richard. *Forging Peace: The Challenge of Central America.* Washington, D.C.: Policy Alternatives for the Caribbean and Central America, 1987.

Galeano, Eduardo. *Memory of Fire: Century of the Wind.* New York: Pantheon Books, 1988.

Hamilton, Nora, Jeffry A. Frieden, Linda Fuller, and Manuel Pastor, Jr., editors. *Crisis in Central America: Regional Dynamics and U.S. Policy in the 1980's.* Boulder: Westview Press, 1988.

Johnson, Paul. *Modern Times: The World from the Twenties to the Eighties.* New York: Perennial Library, Harper and Row, 1983.

Kinzer, Stephen, and Stephen Schlesinger. *Bitter Fruit: The Untold Story of the American Coup in Guatemala.* New York: Anchor Books,1982.

LaFeber, Walter. *Inevitable Revolutions: The United States in Central America.* New York: W. W. Norton and Company, 1984.

Lernoux, Penny. *Cry of the Poor: The Struggle for Human Rights in Latin America — The Catholic Church in Conflict with U.S. Policy.* New York: Penguin Books, 1980.

Lernoux, Penny. *People of God: The Struggle for World Catholicism.* New York: Viking Penguin, Inc., 1989.

Lyon, Peter. *Eisenhower: Portrait of a Hero.* Boston: Little, Brown and Company, 1974.

Martin, Malachi. *The Jesuits: The Society of Jesus and the Betrayal of the Roman Catholic Church.* New York: Touchstone Books, Simon and Schuster, 1987.

Menchu, Rigoberta. *I, Rigoberta Menchu.* New York: New Left Books, 1984.

Nelson-Pallmeyer, Jack. *The Politics of Compassion: Hunger, the Arms Race, and U.S. Policy in Central America.* Maryknoll, N.Y.: Orbis Books, 1988.

Nelson-Pallmeyer, Jack. *War Against the Poor: Low-Intensity Conflict and Christian Faith.* Maryknoll, N.Y.: Orbis Books, 1989.

Schotzko, Philip. *Simple Faith: Stories from Guatemala.* Kansas City: Sheed and Ward, 1989.

Simon, Jean-Marie. *Guatemala: Eternal Spring, Eternal Tyranny.* New York: W. W. Norton and Company, 1987.

Steinbeck, John. *The Grapes of Wrath.* New York: [1939], Penguin Books, 1976.

Summary Report of the Inter-American Dialogue. *The Americas in 1989: Consensus for Action.* Queenstown, MD.: The Aspen Institute, 1989.

Volkman, Ernest and Blaine Baggett. *Secret Intelligence.* New York: Doubleday, 1989.

About the Author

V. David Schwantes is a businessman—a veteran of twenty-five years in corporate America. From 1984 to 1988, he was the president of Vision-Ease, a manufacturing company in the ophthalmic industry. From 1980 to 1984, he was chief financial officer of Medtronic, Inc., a multinational high-technology company in the health care industry. Mr. Schwantes holds an undergraduate degree from Dartmouth College and a master's degree in business and economics from the University of Minnesota. A veteran of the United States Marine Corps and the Marine Corps Reserve, he has served on several hospital, theater, and business boards.